DASH DIET COOKBOOK FOR BEGINNERS 2024

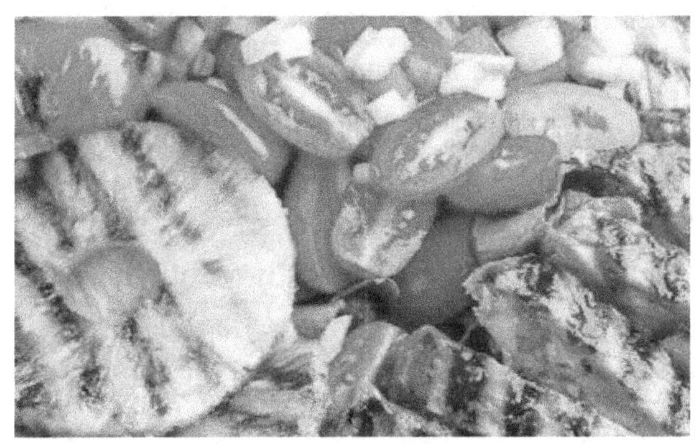

Discover Nourishing Low Sodium Recipes to Lower Your Blood Pressure and Overcome Hypertension, With 30 Day Meal Plan.

Joshua S. Gray

Table of Contents

SCAN THIS CODE TO GAIN ACCESS TO MORE BOOKS BY THE AUTHOR

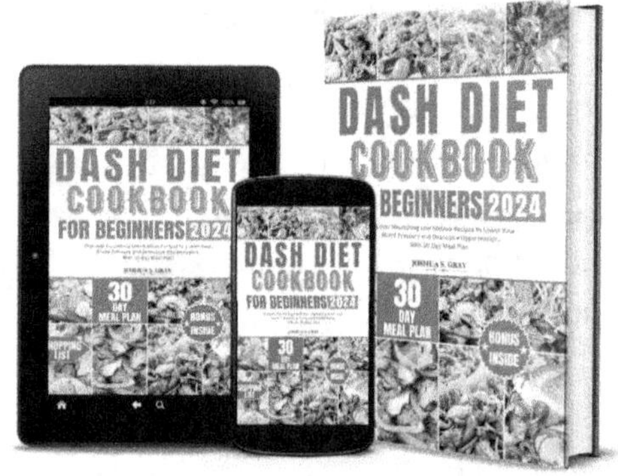

INTRODUCTION

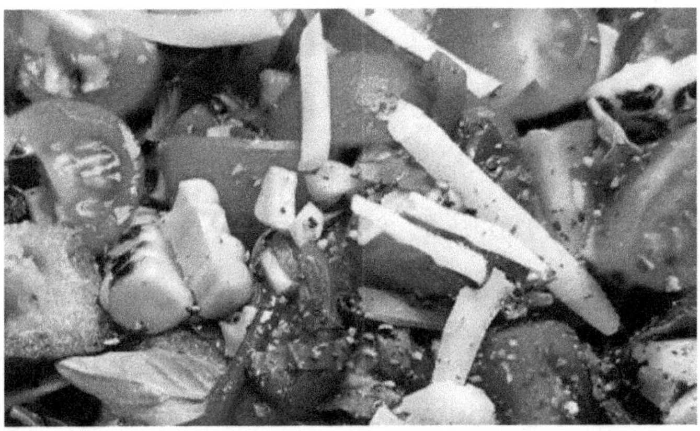

Have you ever wondered why achieving a healthier lifestyle seems like an elusive puzzle?

It's simple to get disoriented in the quest for better health in a world full of fad diets and quick fixes. A lot of people think that the only way to make sense of the maze of wellness is to go overboard or give up on taste. What if I told you there was a way to please your taste buds with a symphony of flavors in addition to achieving vibrant health?

Welcome to the DASH Diet Cookbook For Beginners 2024—a transformative journey to embrace the Dietary Approaches to Stop Hypertension (DASH). It's not just a cookbook; it's your compass to a sustainable and enjoyable approach to health.

Imagine a world where having delicious food and being healthy don't have to conflict, and where meals serve as both nourishment and a celebration of life. Now think about the negative effects that stress, hectic schedules, and processed foods have on our health in today's world. What if there was a way to actually thrive in the face of these obstacles rather than just alleviate them?

We go beyond what is traditionally thought of as dieting with the DASH Diet. It's about abundance in the right decisions, not about deprivation. Imagine enjoying meals that not only tempt your palate but also provide your body with internal nourishment. What if discovering a healthier you is accompanied by vivid colors, alluring scents, and a path to better health?

You will discover a wealth of information within the pages of this cookbook, in addition to recipes. Discover how each component affects your health, the principles underlying the DASH Diet, and how it affects hypertension. With the help of this book, you can begin living a lifestyle that nourishes your body and soul in addition to what you eat.

Feel the resonance of your desire to improve your health, and have faith that this cookbook is your companion on this life-changing journey rather than just a guide. Recognize the difficulties, accept the obstacles, and look forward to a time when meals provide you with energy rather than just nourishment.

Your health is your wealth, and the DASH Diet Cookbook For Beginners 2024 is your ticket to a richer, more vibrant life. Your journey to better health starts with a turn of the page.

CHAPTER 1

What is Dash Diet?

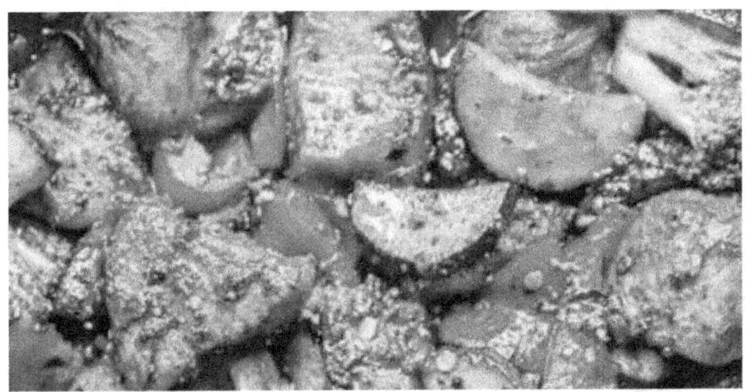

The DASH Diet, or Dietary Approaches to Stop Hypertension, is a scientifically-backed dietary plan designed to prevent and manage hypertension, commonly known as high blood pressure. Developed by the National Heart, Lung, and Blood Institute (NHLBI), the DASH Diet has gained recognition for its effectiveness in promoting heart health and reducing the risk of cardiovascular diseases.

Origins and Purpose

The DASH Diet was introduced in the 1990s in response to the increasing prevalence of hypertension and its association with heart-related issues. It stemmed from the need for a holistic approach to nutrition that could not only address high blood pressure but also contribute to overall cardiovascular well-being. The fundamental premise was to create a dietary pattern that emphasizes nutrient-rich foods while minimizing the intake of sodium, a key contributor to elevated blood pressure.

Core Principles

1. Fruits and Vegetables:

- Central to the DASH Diet is the abundant consumption of fruits and vegetables. These nutrient-dense foods provide essential minerals, antioxidants and vitamins that support overall health. The emphasis on potassium-rich fruits and vegetables helps counteract the effects of sodium.

2. Whole Grains:

- Whole grains, such as brown rice, whole wheat, oats, and quinoa, are integral components of the DASH Diet. They offer fiber, which aids digestion and helps control blood pressure.

3. Lean Proteins:

-        The diet encourages lean protein sources, including poultry, fish, beans, and legumes, while discouraging red meat and processed meats high in saturated fats. This promotes heart-healthy fats and proteins.

4. Dairy or Dairy Alternatives:

-        Low-fat or fat-free dairy products are recommended for their calcium content, essential for bone health. Dairy alternatives, like fortified plant-based milk, can also be incorporated.

5. Nuts, Seeds, and Legumes:

-        Nuts, seeds, and legumes are embraced for their nutritional richness, providing healthy fats, protein, and fiber. They contribute to satiety and overall cardiovascular health.

6. Limited Sodium:

-       A key tenet of the DASH Diet is the reduction of sodium intake. Excessive sodium can lead to fluid retention and elevated blood pressure. Thus, the diet encourages the use of herbs, spices, and other flavorings as alternatives to salt.

7. Moderate Alcohol Consumption:

-       While not a mandatory component, the DASH Diet acknowledges the role of alcohol and advises moderate consumption. If you decide to drink, moderation is defined as having no more than one drink for women and two for men per day.

8. Portion Control:

-       Mindful eating and portion control are emphasized to prevent overconsumption of calories. This aligns with the broader goal of weight management and cardiovascular health.

9. Adaptability:

- One of the strengths of the DASH Diet is its adaptability. It accommodates various dietary preferences, cultural influences, and individual needs, making it accessible to a diverse range of individuals.

10. Scientific Backing:

- The DASH Diet's efficacy is supported by extensive research and clinical studies. It has been shown to significantly lower blood pressure and improve lipid profiles, making it a valuable tool in preventing and managing hypertension.

In essence, the DASH Diet is not just a temporary eating plan; it is a sustainable lifestyle approach that promotes long-term cardiovascular health. Its comprehensive and flexible nature makes it suitable for individuals seeking a balanced and heart-healthy way of eating. Before embarking on any significant dietary changes, consulting with a healthcare professional or registered dietitian is advisable to ensure personalized and safe guidance. The DASH Diet stands as a testament to the profound impact that nutrition can have on overall health and well-being.

Importance of Nutritional Balance and Portion Size

Nutritional balance and portion size play pivotal roles in the effectiveness of the DASH Diet (Dietary Approaches to Stop Hypertension). These two factors are essential components that contribute to the diet's success in promoting heart health, managing blood pressure, and fostering overall well-being. Here's a closer look at the importance of nutritional balance and portion control in the context of the DASH Diet:

1.   **Nutritional Balance:**

a. Macronutrient Distribution:

-       The DASH Diet emphasizes a balanced distribution of macronutrients — carbohydrates, proteins, and fats. This balance is crucial for providing the body with the necessary energy and nutrients for optimal functioning.

b. Heart-Healthy Fats:

-       Prioritizing heart-healthy fats, such as those found in avocados, olive oil, and fatty fish, contributes to overall cardiovascular health. These fats help manage cholesterol levels and support various bodily functions.

c. Adequate Fiber Intake:

-       The diet promotes the consumption of fiber-rich foods, including fruits, vegetables, and whole grains. Adequate fiber intake supports digestive health, helps maintain healthy blood sugar levels, and contributes to a feeling of fullness.

d. Nutrient-Rich Choices:

- Nutrient-rich foods, like fruits, vegetables, nuts, and seeds, are staples of the DASH Diet. These foods provide essential vitamins, minerals, and antioxidants that support overall health and help prevent nutrient deficiencies.

e. Sodium Reduction:

- Balancing the intake of sodium with other electrolytes, such as potassium, is crucial for managing blood pressure. The DASH Diet's focus on potassium-rich foods helps counteract the effects of sodium and supports a healthy balance.

2. Portion Size:

a. Caloric Control:

- Controlling portion sizes is instrumental in managing caloric intake. Maintaining a healthy weight is important for cardiovascular health, and portion control helps prevent overconsumption of calories.

b. Blood Pressure Management:

- Overeating, especially foods high in sodium and saturated fats, can contribute to high blood pressure. Portion control is a key strategy to prevent excessive calorie and sodium intake, supporting blood pressure management.

c. Satiety and Weight Maintenance:

- Eating balanced and appropriately sized meals promotes satiety, preventing excessive snacking and promoting weight maintenance.

Maintaining a healthy weight is a critical factor in preventing and managing hypertension.

d. Mindful Eating:

-        The DASH Diet encourages mindful eating, paying attention to hunger and fullness cues. This practice fosters a healthier relationship with food and helps prevent overeating.

e. Adaptability:

-        Portion control makes the DASH Diet adaptable to individual needs and preferences. It allows individuals to tailor their intake based on factors like age, gender, activity level, and overall health status.

3.   Overall Impact:

a. Comprehensive Heart Health:

-      The combination of nutritional balance and portion control in the DASH Diet contributes to comprehensive heart health. It addresses multiple aspects, including blood pressure management, cholesterol levels, and weight control.

b. Long-Term Sustainability:

-      Nutritional balance and portion control are sustainable practices that can be incorporated into daily life. Unlike fad diets that often rely on extreme restrictions, the DASH Diet's focus on balance and moderation makes it a viable and sustainable long-term approach to eating.

In summary, nutritional balance and portion size are integral aspects of the DASH Diet that work synergistically to promote cardiovascular health. Embracing these principles fosters a sustainable and balanced way of eating, aligning with the broader goal of preventing and managing hypertension and related cardiovascular conditions.

CHAPTER 2

Foods to Limit or Avoid

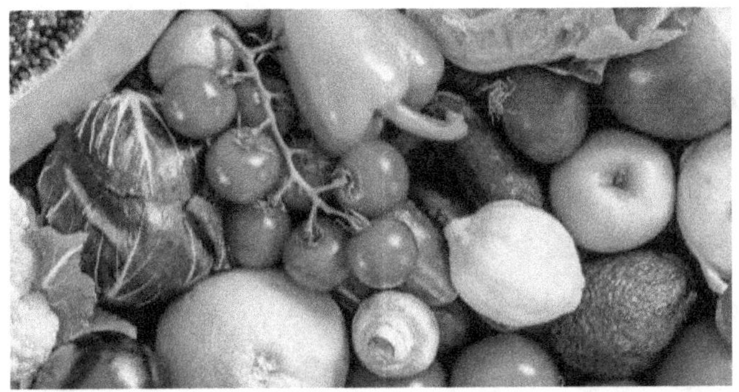

To optimize the benefits of the DASH Diet, it's important to be mindful of certain foods that should be limited or avoided. Here are key categories of foods to restrict in the context of the DASH Diet:

1. **High-Sodium Foods:**

a. **Processed Foods:**

-       Sodium content is high in many packaged and processed foods. This includes canned soups, pre-packaged meals, and processed meats. Choose whole, fresh foods whenever you can.

b. **Fast Food:**

-       Fast food is often laden with sodium. Burgers, fries, and other fast-food items contribute significantly to daily sodium intake. Limiting or avoiding these options is crucial.

c. **Condiments:**

-       High-sodium condiments such as soy sauce, ketchup, and certain salad dressings can contribute to elevated sodium levels. Choose low-sodium alternatives or use them sparingly.

2. Foods High in Saturated Fat:

a. Fatty Meats:

-       Limit your intake of red meats, especially those that are high in fat. Choose lean cuts of meat and poultry or incorporate plant-based protein sources.

b. Full-Fat Dairy:

-       Whole milk, full-fat yogurt, and cheeses can be high in saturated fat. Choose dairy substitutes that are fat-free or low-fat.

c. Processed Snacks:

-       Snack foods like potato chips, crackers, and certain baked goods often contain unhealthy saturated fats. Choose healthier snack options such as nuts or air-popped popcorn.

3.   Added Sugars:

a. Sugary Beverages:

-        Soft drinks, energy drinks, and sugary juices can contribute to excess calorie intake and are associated with various health issues. Choose water, herbal tea, or beverages without added sugars.

b. Sweets and Pastries:

-        Desserts, candies, and pastries often contain added sugars and may be high in unhealthy fats. Choose naturally sweeter options, such as fresh fruit.

4.   **High-Cholesterol Foods:**

a. Organ Meats:

-       Certain organ meats, like liver, are high in cholesterol. Limit the consumption of these foods and choose lean protein sources.

b. Shellfish:

-       Some shellfish, such as shrimp, can be higher in cholesterol. While they can be part of a healthy diet, it's advisable to consume them in moderation.

5.   **Excessive Alcohol:**

a. Moderation is Key:

-       While moderate alcohol consumption may have certain health benefits, excessive alcohol intake can contribute to various health issues, including hypertension. If you decide to drink, make sure you do it in moderation.

6.   Caffeine:

a. Limit Caffeine Intake:

-       While moderate caffeine intake is generally considered safe, excessive consumption can contribute to increased blood pressure in some individuals. Be mindful of your caffeine intake, especially if sensitive to its effects.

7.   Processed Grains:

a. White Bread and Pasta:

-       Refined grains, such as white bread and pasta, lack the fiber and nutrients found in whole grains. Select whole grains such as whole wheat, quinoa, and brown rice.

By being conscious of these categories and making informed choices, individuals can align their eating habits with the principles of the DASH Diet.

Strategies For Successfully Following the Dash Diet

Successfully following the DASH Diet (Dietary Approaches to Stop Hypertension) requires a combination of mindful eating habits, lifestyle adjustments, and strategic planning. Here are strategies to help you adhere to the DASH Diet and promote heart-healthy eating:

1. Understand the Principles:

- Educate Yourself: Familiarize yourself with the key principles of the DASH Diet, which emphasizes fruits, vegetables, lean proteins, whole grains, and low-fat dairy. Understand the recommended daily servings for each food group.

2. Plan Balanced Meals:

-       Meal Prep: Plan your meals in advance, incorporating a balance of fruits, vegetables, lean proteins, and whole grains. Prepare meals in batches to make healthy choices more convenient.

3. Focus on Whole Foods:

-       Select Whole Grains: Make the choice of whole grains like whole wheat, quinoa, and brown rice. When compared to refined grains, these offer more nutrients and fiber.

4. Increase Fruit and Vegetable Intake:

-       Colorful Choices: Include a variety of colorful fruits and vegetables in your meals. Aim to fill half your plate with these nutrient-dense options.

5. Control Portion Sizes:

- Be Mindful: Pay attention to portion sizes to avoid overeating. Reduce the size of your plates to aid in portion control.

6. Monitor Sodium Intake:

- Read Labels: Check food labels for sodium content. Choose low-sodium or no-added-salt versions of products when possible. Limit the use of added salt during cooking.

7. Opt for Lean Proteins:

- Lean Choices: Choose lean protein sources such as poultry, fish, beans, and legumes. Limit red meat intake and opt for healthier cooking methods like grilling or baking.

8. Incorporate Dairy Wisely:

- Choose Low-Fat Dairy: Select low-fat or fat-free dairy products to reduce saturated fat intake. This includes milk, yogurt, and cheese.

9. Snack Smart:

- Healthy Snacks: Keep nutritious snacks on hand, such as fresh fruits, vegetables with hummus, or a handful of nuts. Avoid processed snacks high in sodium and saturated fats.

10. Stay Hydrated:

- Water First: Drink plenty of water throughout the day. Limit sugary beverages and excessive caffeine. Hydration is key to overall health.

11. Gradual Changes:

- Small Steps: Implement changes gradually. Start by making small adjustments to your diet and gradually incorporate more DASH-friendly choices.

12. Seek Support:

- Community or Family Involvement: If possible, involve family members or friends in your DASH Diet journey. Having a support system can make the process more enjoyable and sustainable.

13. Mindful Eating:

- Savor Your Meals: Eat mindfully, savoring each bite. Avoid distractions like television or phones during meals to promote mindful eating.

14. Regular Physical Activity:

- Exercise Routine: Combine the DASH Diet with regular physical activity. Aim for 150 minutes or more a week of moderate-to-intense exercise.

15. Track Progress:

-        Keep a Food Journal: Consider keeping a food journal to track your meals, snacks, and overall food choices. You can spot trends and maintain accountability by doing this.

16. Consult a Professional:

-        Registered Dietitian or Healthcare Provider: If possible, consult with a registered dietitian or healthcare professional for personalized guidance and support.

Adhering to the DASH Diet is a lifestyle choice that can lead to long-term health benefits. By incorporating these strategies into your routine, you can successfully follow the DASH Diet and support your overall well-being.

CHAPTER 3

Shopping List

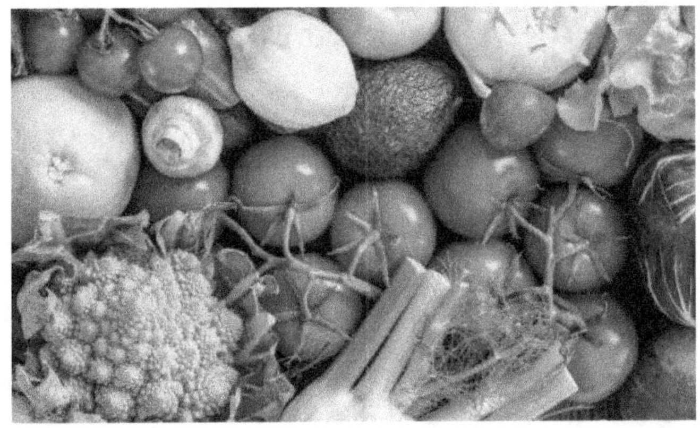

Creating a shopping list for the DASH Diet involves selecting a variety of nutrient-dense foods that align with the principles of the diet. Here's a sample shopping list to guide you:

1. Fruits (e.g., apples, berries, oranges, bananas)

2. Vegetables (e.g., leafy greens, broccoli, carrots, bell peppers)

3. Avocados

4. Berries (blueberries, strawberries, raspberries)

5. Tomatoes

Whole Grains:

6. Brown rice

7. Quinoa

8. Oats (steel-cut or rolled oats)

9. Whole wheat pasta

10. Barley

Lean Proteins:

11. Skinless poultry (chicken or turkey breast)

12. Fish (salmon, trout, tuna)

13. Lean cuts of beef or pork

14. Beans and legumes (black beans, lentils, chickpeas)

15. Tofu or tempeh

Dairy:

16. Low-fat or fat-free milk

17. Greek yogurt

18. Cottage cheese

19. Reduced-fat cheese

Nuts and Seeds:

20. Almonds

21. Walnuts

22. Chia seeds

23. Flaxseeds

Healthy Fats:

24. Olive oil

25. Avocado oil

26. Nuts and nut butter

Herbs and Spices:

27. Fresh herbs (cilantro, basil, parsley)

28. Spices (cumin, turmeric, garlic powder)

Low-Sodium Products:

29. Low-sodium canned beans and vegetables

30. Low-sodium broth or stock

Beverages:

31. Water

32. Herbal teas

33. Freshly squeezed juices (without added sugar)

Snacks:

34. Hummus

35. Whole-grain crackers

36. Popcorn (unsalted)

37. Fresh fruit for snacking

Miscellaneous:

38. Eggs

39. Dark chocolate (in moderation)

40. DASH-friendly condiments (mustard, vinegar)

Optional:

41. Whole-grain bread

42. Poultry or plant-based burgers

43. Greek yogurt-based dressing

Remember to adapt the list based on your personal preferences and dietary needs. Additionally, always check food labels for sodium content, and choose low-sodium or no-added-salt versions of products when available. Aim to prioritize whole, unprocessed foods to support the DASH Diet's heart-healthy principles.

Essential Exercises That Complement Dash Diet

The DASH Diet (Dietary Approaches to Stop Hypertension) emphasizes a balanced and heart-healthy approach to eating, but incorporating regular exercise further enhances its benefits. Here are essential exercises that complement the DASH Diet:

1. Brisk Walking:

- Duration: Try to get 150 minutes or more a week of aerobic activity at a moderate level.

- Benefits: Brisk walking is accessible, low-impact, and an excellent cardiovascular exercise that supports heart health.

2. Cycling:

- Outdoor or Stationary Bike: Cycling is a low-impact exercise that improves cardiovascular fitness.

- Duration: Include cycling sessions in your routine for at least 30 minutes several times a week.

3. Swimming:

- Full-Body Workout: Swimming engages multiple muscle groups and is easy on the joints.

- Benefits: Regular swimming supports cardiovascular health and overall fitness.

4. Strength Training:

- Bodyweight Exercises: Add planks, push-ups, lunges, and squats.

- Resistance Training: Use resistance bands or weights to build muscle strength.

- Benefits: Strength training enhances metabolism, supports weight management, and improves overall strength.

5. Yoga:

- Flexibility and Mindfulness: Yoga combines flexibility exercises with mindfulness.

- Benefits: Reduces stress, improves flexibility, and enhances overall well-being.

6. High-Intensity Interval Training (HIIT):

- Interval Workouts: Alternating between short bursts of intense exercise and periods of rest.

- Benefits: Efficient for burning calories, improving cardiovascular fitness, and promoting weight loss.

7. Elliptical Training:

- Low-Impact Cardio: Elliptical machines provide a full-body workout with minimal impact on joints.

- Benefits: Supports cardiovascular health and is gentle on the joints.

8. Outdoor Activities:

- Hiking: Engage in nature by going for hikes, which offer cardiovascular benefits.

- Gardening: Gardening is a physical activity that contributes to overall well-being.

9. Dancing:

- Enjoyable Cardio: Dancing is a fun way to get your heart rate up.

- Benefits: Promotes cardiovascular health and can be a social activity.

10. Group Fitness Classes:

- Community Engagement: Joining group classes like aerobics or spin can provide motivation.

- Benefits: Group workouts offer social interaction and support.

11. Tai Chi:

- Gentle Movements: Tai Chi combines gentle movements with deep breathing.

- Benefits: Enhances balance, flexibility, and reduces stress.

12. Pilates:

- Core Strengthening: Pilates focuses on core strength and overall body conditioning.

- Benefits: Improves flexibility, posture, and core stability.

13. Mindful Walking:

- Mind-Body Connection: Combine walking with mindfulness practices for a holistic approach.

- Benefits: Reduces stress and enhances the mental well-being component of the DASH Diet.

14. Consultation with a Fitness Professional:

- Personalized Guidance: Consider consulting with a fitness professional for a personalized exercise plan.

- Benefits: Ensures that your exercise routine aligns with your fitness goals and health status.

Always consult with your healthcare provider before starting a new exercise program, especially if you have existing health conditions. Combining the DASH Diet with regular exercise contributes to overall cardiovascular health, weight management, and improved well-being.

CHAPTER 4

Breakfast Recipes

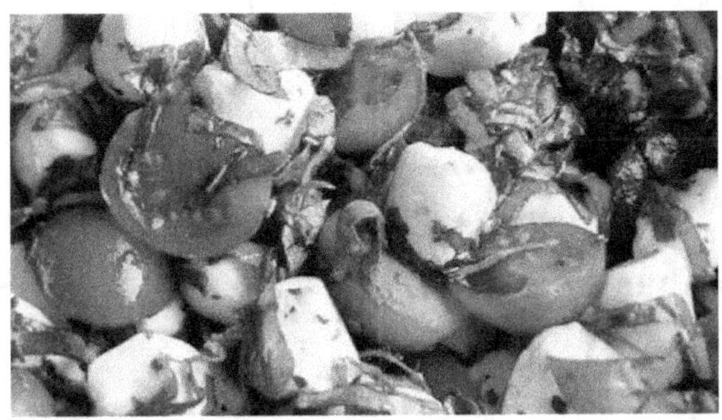

1. Blueberry Oatmeal

Ingredients:

- 1 cup rolled oats

- 1 cup blueberries (fresh or frozen)

- 1 tablespoon honey

- 1 cup skim milk

Preparation:

1. Cook 1 cup of rolled oats with 1 cup of skim milk according to package instructions.

2. Stir in 1 cup of blueberries and 1 tablespoon of honey.

3. Cook until oats are tender.

Nutritional Information (per serving):

- Calories: 300

- Protein: 10g

- Carbohydrates: 50g

- Fiber: 8g

- Potassium: 300mg

Cooking Time: 10 minutes

2. Scrambled Egg and Vegetables

Ingredients:

- 2 eggs, beaten

- ½ cup diced bell peppers

- ½ cup cherry tomatoes, halved

- ¼ cup chopped spinach

- Salt and pepper to taste

Preparation:

1. In a non-stick pan, cook ½ cup each of diced bell peppers and cherry tomatoes until softened.

2. Add ¼ cup chopped spinach.

3. Pour 2 beaten eggs over the vegetables and scramble until cooked.

4. Season with pepper and salt.

Nutritional Information (per serving):

- Calories: 220

- Protein: 14g

- Carbohydrates: 10g

- Fiber: 3g

- Potassium: 250mg

Cooking Time: 15 minutes

3. Avocado and Egg Toast

Ingredients:

- 1 slice whole-grain bread

- ½ avocado, sliced

- 1 poached egg

- Salt and pepper to taste

Preparation:

1. Toast 1 slice of whole-grain bread.

2. Top with ½ sliced avocado and 1 poached egg.

3. Season with pepper and salt.

Nutritional Information (per serving):

- Calories: 280

- Protein: 12g

- Carbohydrates: 20g

- Fiber: 8g

- Potassium: 400mg

Cooking Time: 10 minutes

4. Veggie Omelet

Ingredients:

- 2 eggs, beaten
- ¼ cup diced onions
- ¼ cup diced bell peppers
- ¼ cup chopped mushrooms
- ¼ cup shredded low-fat cheese

Preparation:

1. In a non-stick pan, cook ¼ cup each of diced onions, bell peppers, and mushrooms until tender.

2. Pour 2 beaten eggs over the vegetables and cook until set.

3. Sprinkle with ¼ cup shredded low-fat cheese on one side and fold.

Nutritional Information (per serving):

- Calories: 250

- Protein: 15g

- Carbohydrates: 10g

- Fiber: 3g

- Potassium: 300mg

Cooking Time: 10 minutes

5. Pineapple Coconut Smoothie

Ingredients:

- 1 cup fresh pineapple chunks
- ½ cup coconut milk
- ½ cup Greek yogurt
- Ice cubes

Preparation:

1. Blend 1 cup fresh pineapple chunks, ½ cup coconut milk, and ½ cup Greek yogurt until smooth.

2. Add ice cubes and blend again.

Nutritional Information (per serving):

- Calories: 200

- Protein: 8g

- Carbohydrates: 25g

- Fiber: 2g

- Potassium: 300mg

Prep Time: 5 minutes

6. Chia Seed Pudding

Ingredients:

- 2 tablespoons chia seeds

- ½ cup almond milk

- ½ teaspoon vanilla extract

- Fresh berries for topping

Preparation:

1. In a jar, mix 2 tablespoons chia seeds, ½ cup almond milk, and ½ teaspoon vanilla extract.

2. Refrigerate overnight.

3. Top with fresh berries before serving.

Nutritional Information (per serving):

- Calories: 180

- Protein: 5g

- Carbohydrates: 15g

- Fiber: 10g

- Potassium: 150mg

Prep Time: 5 minutes + Overnight refrigeration

7. Quinoa Breakfast Porridge

Ingredients:

- ½ cup cooked quinoa

- ½ cup almond milk

- 1 tablespoon honey

- Sliced banana for topping

Preparation:

1. Heat ½ cup cooked quinoa with ½ cup almond milk.

2. Stir in 1 tablespoon honey.

3. Top with sliced banana.

Nutritional Information (per serving):

- Calories: 220

- Protein: 6g

- Carbohydrates: 40g

- Fiber: 5g

- Potassium: 200mg

Cooking Time: 10 minutes

8. Oat Bran with Berries

- ½ cup oat bran

- 1 cup mixed berries

- 1 tablespoon flaxseeds

- ¼ cup skim milk

Preparation:

1. Cook ½ cup oat bran with ¼ cup skim milk according to package instructions.

2. Top with 1 cup mixed berries and 1 tablespoon flaxseeds.

Nutritional Information (per serving):

- Calories: 240

- Protein: 7g

- Carbohydrates: 45g

- Fiber: 8g

- Potassium: 250mg

Cooking Time: 5 minutes

9. Cottage Cheese with Fresh Fruit

Ingredients:

- ½ cup low-fat cottage cheese
- ½ cup diced fresh fruit (e.g., melon, berries)
- 1 tablespoon chopped nuts (optional)

Preparation:

1. Mix ½ cup low-fat cottage cheese with ½ cup diced fresh fruit.

2. Sprinkle with 1 tablespoon chopped nuts if desired.

Nutritional Information (per serving):

- Calories: 180

- Protein: 15g

- Carbohydrates: 20g

- Fiber: 3g

- Potassium: 200mg

Prep Time: 5 minutes

10. Sweet Potato Hash Browns

Ingredients:

- 1 medium sweet potato, grated

- 1 tablespoon olive oil

- ½ teaspoon paprika

- Salt and pepper to taste

Preparation:

1. Squeeze excess moisture from 1 medium grated sweet potato.

2. Heat 1 tablespoon olive oil in a pan, add sweet potato, paprika, salt, and pepper. Cook until crispy.

Nutritional Information (per serving):

- Calories: 180

- Protein: 2g

- Carbohydrates: 25g

- Fiber: 4g

- Potassium: 400mg

Cooking Time: 15 minutes

CHAPTER 5

Lunch Recipes

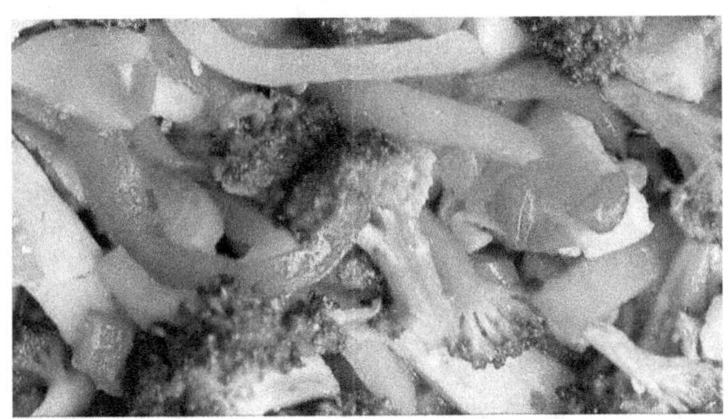

1. Chicken and Vegetable Stir Fry

Ingredients:

- 1 cup diced chicken breast

- 1 cup broccoli florets

- ½ cup sliced bell peppers

- ½ cup snap peas

- 1 tablespoon low-sodium soy sauce

Preparation:

1. Stir fry 1 cup diced chicken breast until cooked.

2. Add 1 cup broccoli, ½ cup bell peppers, and ½ cup snap peas.

3. Drizzle with 1 tablespoon low-sodium soy sauce.

Nutritional Information (per serving):

- Calories: 300
- Protein: 25g
- Carbohydrates: 15g
- Fiber: 5g
- Potassium: 400mg

Cooking Time: 15 minutes

2. Turkey and Vegetable Chili

Ingredients:

- 1 cup ground turkey

- 1 can (15 oz) of drained kidney beans

- 1 can (15 oz) of tomatoes (diced)

- ½ cup diced onions

- ½ cup diced bell peppers

- 1 tablespoon chili powder

Preparation:

1. Brown 1 cup ground turkey in a pot.

2. Add 1 can kidney beans, 1 can diced tomatoes, ½ cup onions, ½ cup bell peppers, and 1 tablespoon chili powder.

3. Simmer until flavors meld.

Nutritional Information (per serving):

- Calories: 320

- Protein: 20g

- Carbohydrates: 30g

- Fiber: 10g

- Potassium: 500mg

Cooking Time: 30 minutes

3. Grilled Lemon Herb Chicken

Ingredients:

- 2 boneless, skinless chicken breasts

- 1 lemon (juiced)

- 2 tablespoons olive oil

- 1 teaspoon dried herbs like thyme, oregano, rosemary

- Salt and pepper to taste

Preparation:

1. Marinate 2 chicken breasts in a mixture of lemon juice, olive oil, dried herbs, salt, and pepper.

2. Grill until fully cooked.

Nutritional Information (per serving):

- Calories: 250

- Protein: 30g

- Carbohydrates: 2g

- Fiber: 0g

- Potassium: 300mg

Cooking Time: 20 minutes

4. Greek Style Quinoa Salad

Ingredients:

- 1 cup cooked quinoa
- ½ cup cherry tomatoes, halved
- ¼ cup diced cucumber
- ¼ cup crumbled feta cheese
- Kalamata olives (to taste)
- 2 tablespoons olive oil
- 1 tablespoon red wine vinegar
- Fresh oregano (optional)

Preparation:

1. Mix 1 cup cooked quinoa with cherry tomatoes, cucumber, feta cheese, and Kalamata olives.

2. Mix red wine vinegar and olive oil for dressing.

3. Garnish with fresh oregano if desired.

Nutritional Information (per serving):

- Calories: 350

- Protein: 10g

- Carbohydrates: 30g

- Fiber: 5g

- Potassium: 200mg

Prep Time: 15 minutes

5. Grilled Chicken Quinoa Salad

Ingredients:

- 1 cup cooked quinoa

- 1 grilled chicken breast, sliced

- ½ cup cherry tomatoes, halved

- ¼ cup sliced cucumbers

- ¼ cup crumbled feta cheese

- 2 tablespoons balsamic vinaigrette

Preparation:

1. Assemble 1 cup cooked quinoa, grilled chicken slices, cherry tomatoes, cucumber, and feta cheese.

2. Drizzle with balsamic vinaigrette.

Nutritional Information (per serving):

- Calories: 380

- Protein: 25g

- Carbohydrates: 30g

- Fiber: 5g

- Potassium: 250mg

Prep Time: 20 minutes

6. Baked Salmon with Lemon and Dill

Ingredients:

- 2 salmon fillets

- 1 lemon (sliced)

- Fresh dill (to taste)

- Salt and pepper to taste

Preparation:

1. Place 2 salmon fillets on a baking sheet.

2. Top with lemon slices and fresh dill.

3. Bake until salmon is cooked through.

Nutritional Information (per serving):

- Calories: 300

- Protein: 30g

- Carbohydrates: 2g

- Fiber: 0g

- Potassium: 500mg

Cooking Time: 15 minutes

7. Chicken Curry with Vegetables

- 1 cup cooked chicken breast, diced

- ½ cup broccoli florets

- ½ cup cauliflower florets

- ½ cup carrots, sliced

- ½ cup green beans, chopped

- ½ cup light coconut milk

- 1 tablespoon curry powder

Preparation:

1. Stir-fry cooked chicken, broccoli, cauliflower, carrots, and green beans.

2. Add light coconut milk and curry powder. Simmer until vegetables are tender.

Nutritional Information (per serving):

- Calories: 280

- Protein: 25g

- Carbohydrates: 15g

- Fiber: 5g

- Potassium: 400mg

Cooking Time: 20 minutes

8. Veggie and Hummus Wrap

Ingredients:

- 1 whole-grain wrap

- 2 tablespoons hummus

-½ cup mixed veggies (bell peppers, cucumber, lettuce)

- ¼ cup shredded carrots

Preparation:

1. Spread hummus on a whole-grain wrap.

2. Fill with mixed veggies and shredded carrots.

Nutritional Information (per serving):

- Calories: 250

- Protein: 8g

- Carbohydrates: 35g

- Fiber: 8g

- Potassium: 300mg

Prep Time: 10 minutes

9. Mediterranean Quinoa Salad

Ingredients:

- 1 cup cooked quinoa

- ½ cup cherry tomatoes, halved

- ¼ cup diced cucumber

- ¼ cup Kalamata olives

- 2 tablespoons feta cheese

- 1 tablespoon olive oil

- 1 tablespoon red wine vinegar

Preparation:

1. Combine cooked quinoa, cherry tomatoes, cucumber, Kalamata olives, and feta cheese.

2. Mix red wine vinegar and olive oil for dressing.

- Calories: 340

- Protein: 10g

- Carbohydrates: 30g

- Fiber: 5g

- Potassium: 200mg

Prep Time: 15 minutes

10. Grilled Shrimp and Vegetable Kabobs

Ingredients:

- ½ pound of peeled and deveined shrimp

- ½ cup cherry tomatoes

- ½ cup of chopped bell peppers

- ½ cup finely chopped red onion

- ¼ cup pineapple chunks

- 1 tablespoon olive oil

- Lemon wedges (for serving)

Preparation:

1. Thread shrimp, cherry tomatoes, bell peppers, red onion, and pineapple onto skewers.

2. Brush with olive oil and grill until shrimp is opaque.

Nutritional Information (per serving):

- Calories: 280

- Protein: 20g

- Carbohydrates: 20g

- Fiber: 4g

- Potassium: 350mg

Cooking Time: 10 minutes

CHAPTER 6

Dinner Recipes

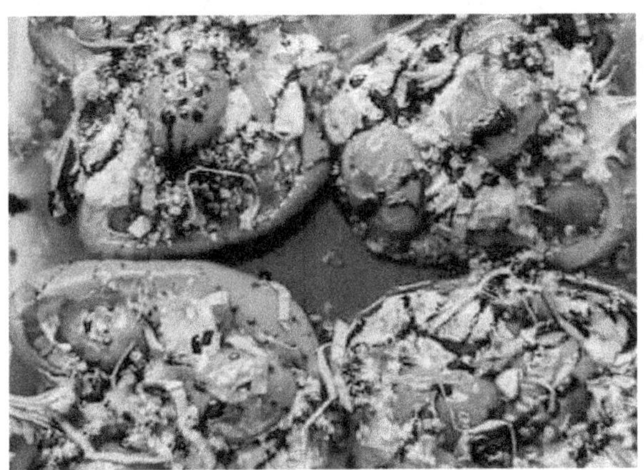

1. Quinoa Stuffed Bell Pepper

Ingredients:

- 4 bell peppers

- 1 cup cooked quinoa

- ½ lb lean ground turkey

- ½ cup black beans, drained and rinsed

- ½ cup corn kernels

- 1 cup diced tomatoes

- 1 teaspoon cumin

- Salt and pepper to taste

Preparation:

1. Cut bell peppers in half and remove seeds.

2. In a bowl, mix cooked quinoa, browned ground turkey, black beans, corn, diced tomatoes, cumin, salt, and pepper.

3. Stuff bell peppers with the mixture.

4. Bake until peppers are tender.

Nutritional Information (per serving):

- Calories: 300

- Protein: 20g

- Carbohydrates: 40g

- Fiber: 8g

- Potassium: 500mg

Cooking Time: 25 minutes

2. Lemon Herb Grilled Chicken Breast

Ingredients:

- 2 boneless, skinless chicken breasts

- 1 lemon (juiced)

- 2 tablespoons olive oil

- 1 teaspoon dried herbs like thyme, oregano, rosemary

- Salt and pepper to taste

Preparation:

1. Marinate chicken breasts in a mixture of lemon juice, olive oil, dried herbs, salt, and pepper.

2. Grill until fully cooked.

Nutritional Information (per serving):

- Calories: 250

- Protein: 30g

- Carbohydrates: 2g

- Fiber: 0g

- Potassium: 300mg

Cooking Time: 20 minutes

3. Baked Cod with Roasted Vegetables

Ingredients:

- 2 cod fillets

- 1 cup cherry tomatoes, halved

- ½ cup zucchini, sliced

- ½ cup bell peppers, sliced

- 1 tablespoon olive oil

- Lemon wedges

Preparation:

1. Place cod fillets on a baking sheet.

2. Surround with cherry tomatoes, zucchini, and bell peppers.

3. Drizzle with olive oil and bake until fish flakes easily.

- Calories: 280

- Protein: 25g

- Carbohydrates: 10g

- Fiber: 3g

- Potassium: 400mg

Cooking Time: 20 minutes

4. Chickpea and Vegetable Curry

Ingredients:

- 1 can (15 oz) chickpeas, drained

- 1 cup cauliflower florets

- ½ cup peas

- ½ cup carrots, sliced

- ½ cup bell peppers, diced

- 1 can (15 oz) chopped tomatoes

- ½ cup light coconut milk

- 1 tablespoon curry powder

Preparation:

1. In a pot, combine chickpeas, cauliflower, peas, carrots, bell peppers, diced tomatoes, coconut milk, and curry powder.

2. Simmer until vegetables are tender.

Nutritional Information (per serving):

- Calories: 320

- Protein: 15g

- Carbohydrates: 50g

- Fiber: 12g

- Potassium: 600mg

Cooking Time: 30 minutes

5. Caprese Stuffed Chicken Breast

Ingredients:

- 2 boneless, skinless chicken breasts

- ½ cup cherry tomatoes, sliced

- ¼ cup fresh mozzarella, diced

- Fresh basil leaves

- Balsamic glaze

Preparation:

1. Make a pocket in each of the chicken breasts.

2. Stuff with cherry tomatoes, mozzarella, and basil.

3. Grill the chicken until it's thoroughly cooked.

4. Drizzle with balsamic glaze.

Nutritional Information (per serving):

- Calories: 280

- Protein: 30g

- Carbohydrates: 4g

- Fiber: 1g

- Potassium: 350mg

Cooking Time: 25 minutes

6. Baked Zucchini Boats with Ground Turkey

Ingredients:

- 4 zucchinis, halved lengthwise

- ½ lb lean ground turkey

- ½ cup onion, diced

- ½ cup bell peppers, diced

- 1 cup tomato sauce

- 1 teaspoon Italian seasoning

- Salt and pepper to taste

Preparation:

1. Scoop out the center of zucchinis to create boats.

2. In a skillet, brown ground turkey with onion and bell peppers.

3. Stir in tomato sauce, Italian seasoning, salt, and pepper.

4. Fill zucchini boats with the turkey mixture.

5. Bake until zucchini is tender.

Nutritional Information (per serving):

- Calories: 260

- Protein: 25g

- Carbohydrates: 20g

- Fiber: 6g

- Potassium: 450mg

Cooking Time: 30 minutes

7. Spicy Shrimp Stir Fry with Brown Rice

Ingredients:

- ½ pound of peeled and deveined shrimp
- 1 cup broccoli florets
- ½ cup snap peas
- ½ cup carrots, julienned
- 1 tablespoon soy sauce
- 1 teaspoon Sriracha
- 2 cups cooked brown rice

Preparation:

1. In a wok, stir fry shrimp, broccoli, snap peas, and carrots.
2. Mix in soy sauce and Sriracha.
3. Serve over cooked brown rice.

Nutritional Information (per serving):

- Calories: 290

- Protein: 20g

- Carbohydrates: 45g

- Fiber: 6g

- Potassium: 300mg

Cooking Time: 15 minutes

8. Italian Herb Grilled Pork Chops

Ingredients:

- 2 bone-in pork chops

- 1 tablespoon olive oil

- 1 teaspoon dried Italian herbs

- ½ teaspoon garlic powder

- Salt and pepper to taste

Preparation:

1. Rub pork chops with olive oil, Italian herbs, garlic powder, salt, and pepper.

2. Grill until fully cooked.

Nutritional Information (per serving):

- Calories: 280

- Protein: 25g

- Carbohydrates: 0g

- Fiber: 0g

- Potassium: 350mg

Cooking Time: 20 minutes

9. Mexican Quinoa Skillet

Ingredients:

- 1 cup cooked quinoa

- ½ lb ground chicken

- 1 cup of rinsed and drained black beans

- 1 cup corn kernels

- ½ cup bell peppers, diced

- 1 teaspoon chili powder

- ½ teaspoon cumin

- Salt and pepper to taste

Preparation:

1. In a skillet, brown ground chicken.

2. Stir in cooked quinoa, black beans, corn, bell peppers, chili powder, cumin, salt, and pepper.

3. Cook until heated through.

Nutritional Information (per serving):

- Calories: 310

- Protein: 25g

- Carbohydrates: 45g

- Fiber: 8g

- Potassium: 500mg

Cooking Time: 25 minutes

10. Thai Red Curry with Tofu and Vegetables

Ingredients:

- 1 block firm tofu, cubed

- 1 cup broccoli florets

- ½ cup red bell peppers, sliced

- ½ cup snap peas

- 1 (14-ounce) can of coconut milk

- 2 tablespoons Thai red curry paste

- 1 tablespoon soy sauce

- Fresh cilantro for garnish

Preparation:

1. In a pot, combine tofu, broccoli, bell peppers, snap peas, coconut milk, red curry paste, and soy sauce.

2. Simmer until vegetables are tender.

3. Garnish with fresh cilantro.

Nutritional Information (per serving):

- Calories: 320

- Protein: 15g

- Carbohydrates: 20g

- Fiber: 5g

- Potassium: 400mg

Cooking Time: 30 minutes

CHAPTER 7

Fish and Seafood Recipes

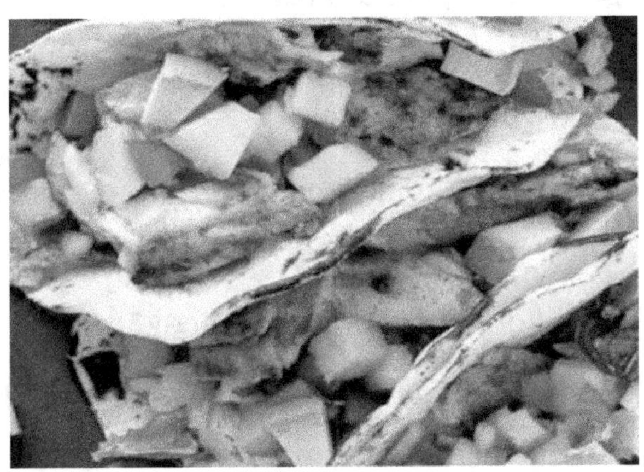

1. Tilapia Tacos with Mango Salsa

Ingredients:

- 4 tilapia fillets

- 8 small whole-grain tortillas

- 1 cup mango, diced

- ½ cup red onion, finely chopped

- ¼ cup fresh cilantro, chopped

- 1 jalapeño, seeded and minced

- 1 tablespoon lime juice

- 1 teaspoon ground cumin

- Salt and pepper to taste

Preparation:

1. Season tilapia fillets with cumin, salt, and pepper.

2. Grill or bake tilapia until cooked.

3. In a bowl, combine mango, red onion, cilantro, jalapeño, and lime juice to make salsa.

4. Assemble tacos with tilapia and mango salsa.

Nutritional Information (per serving):

- Calories: 280

- Protein: 30g

- Carbohydrates: 30g

- Fiber: 5g

- Potassium: 450mg

Cooking Time: 20 minutes

2. Baked Cod with Lemon Pepper Sauce

Ingredients:

- 4 cod fillets

- 2 tablespoons olive oil

- 2 tablespoons lemon juice

- 1 teaspoon lemon zest

- 1 teaspoon black pepper

- ½ teaspoon garlic powder

- Fresh parsley for garnish

Preparation:

1. Preheat the oven and place cod fillets on a baking sheet.

2. In a bowl, mix olive oil, lemon juice, lemon zest, black pepper, and garlic powder.

3. Brush the cod fillets with the lemon pepper mixture.

4. Bake until cod is flaky.

5. Garnish with fresh parsley.

Nutritional Information (per serving):

- Calories: 220

- Protein: 25g

- Carbohydrates: 1g

- Fiber: 0g

- Potassium: 400mg

Cooking Time: 15 minutes

3. Lemon Garlic Shrimp and Broccoli Stir Fry

Ingredients:

- 1 pound of peeled and deveined shrimp

- 3 cups broccoli florets

- 3 cloves garlic, minced

- 2 tablespoons olive oil

- 2 tablespoons lemon juice

- 1 teaspoon lemon zest

- Salt and pepper to taste

Preparation:

1. In a skillet, heat olive oil and sauté garlic until fragrant.

2. Add shrimp and cook until pink.

3. Stir in broccoli, lemon juice, and lemon zest.

4. Cook until broccoli is tender.

5. Season with salt and pepper.

Nutritional Information (per serving):

- Calories: 250

- Protein: 30g

- Carbohydrates: 8g

- Fiber: 3g

- Potassium: 500mg

Cooking Time: 20 minutes

4. Grilled Swordfish with Herb Butter

- 4 swordfish steaks

- 2 tablespoons unsalted butter, melted

- 1 tablespoon fresh parsley, chopped

- 1 tablespoon fresh dill, chopped

- 1 teaspoon lemon juice

- Salt and pepper to taste

Preparation:

1. Preheat the grill.

2. Season swordfish steaks with salt and pepper.

3. Grill swordfish until cooked.

4. In a bowl, mix melted butter, parsley, dill, and lemon juice.

5. Drizzle herb butter over grilled swordfish.

Nutritional Information (per serving):

- Calories: 300

- Protein: 25g

- Carbohydrates: 0g

- Fiber: 0g

- Potassium: 450mg

Cooking Time: 15 minutes

5. Tuna Salad Lettuce Wraps

Ingredients:

- 2 cans tuna, drained
- ¼ cup mayonnaise
- 1 celery stalk, finely chopped
- ¼ cup red onion, finely chopped
- 1 teaspoon Dijon mustard
- Salt and pepper to taste
- Lettuce leaves for wrapping

Preparation:

1. In a bowl, mix tuna, mayonnaise, celery, red onion, Dijon mustard, salt, and pepper.
2. Spoon tuna salad onto lettuce leaves.
3. Wrap and secure with toothpicks.

Nutritional Information (per serving):

- Calories: 200

- Protein: 20g

- Carbohydrates: 2g

- Fiber: 1g

- Potassium: 300mg

Preparation Time: 10 minutes

6. Shrimp and Quinoa Stir Fry

Ingredients:

- 1 pound of peeled and deveined shrimp

- 1 cup quinoa, cooked

- 1 cup broccoli florets

- 1 bell pepper, sliced

- 2 tablespoons low-sodium soy sauce

- 1 tablespoon sesame oil

- 1 teaspoon ginger, minced

- 2 cloves garlic, minced

Preparation:

1. In a wok, heat sesame oil and sauté garlic and ginger.

2. Add shrimp and cook until pink.

3. Stir in cooked quinoa, broccoli, and bell pepper.

4. Add soy sauce and toss until well combined.

Nutritional Information (per serving):

- Calories: 320

- Protein: 25g

- Carbohydrates: 35g

- Fiber: 5g

- Potassium: 400mg

Cooking Time: 20 minutes

7. Lemon Herb Baked Tilapia

Ingredients:

- 4 tilapia fillets

- 2 tablespoons olive oil

- 2 tablespoons lemon juice

- 1 teaspoon dried thyme

- 1 teaspoon dried rosemary

- Salt and pepper to taste

Preparation:

1. Preheat the oven and place tilapia fillets on a baking sheet.

2. In a small bowl, mix olive oil, lemon juice, thyme, rosemary, salt, and pepper.

3. Brush the tilapia fillets with the lemon herb mixture.

4. Bake until tilapia is cooked through.

Nutritional Information (per serving):

- Calories: 180

- Protein: 25g

- Carbohydrates: 0g

- Fiber: 0g

- Potassium: 350mg

Cooking Time: 15 minutes

8. Shrimp and Vegetable Skewers

Ingredients:

- 1 pound of peeled and deveined shrimp
- Cherry tomatoes
- Bell peppers, assorted colors
- Zucchini, sliced
- Red onion, sliced
- Olive oil
- Paprika, salt, garlic powder and pepper

Preparation:

1. Preheat the grill.
2. Thread shrimp and vegetables onto skewers.
3. Brush with olive oil and sprinkle with garlic powder, paprika, salt, and pepper.
4. Grill until shrimp is cooked and vegetables are tender.

Nutritional Information (per serving):

- Calories: 220

- Protein: 20g

- Carbohydrates: 10g

- Fiber: 3g

- Potassium: 400mg

Cooking Time: 15 minutes

9. Grilled Vegetable and Halloumi Skewers

Ingredients:

- Halloumi cheese, cubed

- Cherry tomatoes

- Red and yellow bell peppers, cut into chunks

- Red onion, cut into wedges

- Zucchini, sliced

- Olive oil

- Lemon juice

- Fresh herbs (rosemary, thyme)

- Salt and pepper to taste

Preparation:

1. Preheat the grill.

2. Thread halloumi and vegetables onto skewers.

3. Mix olive oil, lemon juice, herbs, salt, and pepper in a bowl.

4. Brush skewers with the mixture and grill until halloumi is golden.

Nutritional Information (per serving):

- Calories: 250
- Protein: 15g
- Carbohydrates: 10g
- Fiber: 3g
- Potassium: 300mg

Cooking Time: 10 minutes

10. Baked Lemon Herb Haddock

Ingredients:

- 4 haddock fillets
- 2 tablespoons olive oil
- 1 lemon, sliced
- 1 teaspoon dried oregano
- 1 teaspoon dried thyme
- Salt and pepper to taste

Preparation:

1. Preheat the oven and place haddock fillets on a baking sheet.

2. Drizzle olive oil over the fillets and season with oregano, thyme, salt, and pepper.

3. Place lemon slices on top of the fillets.

4. Bake until haddock is flaky.

- Calories: 180

- Protein: 25g

- Carbohydrates: 1g

- Fiber: 0g

- Potassium: 300mg

Cooking Time: 15 minutes

CHAPTER 8

Snack Recipes

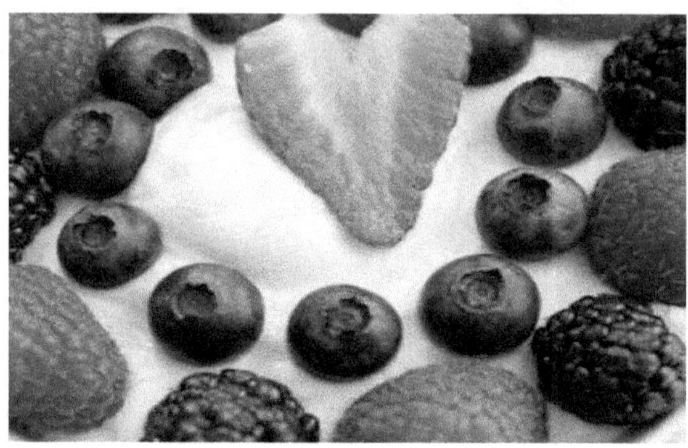

1. Greek Yogurt with Berries

Ingredients:

- 1 cup Greek yogurt

- Mixed berries (strawberries, blueberries, raspberries)

- Honey (optional)

Preparation:

1. Spoon Greek yogurt into a bowl.

2. Top with mixed berries.

3. Drizzle with honey if desired.

Nutritional Information (per serving):

- Calories: 150

- Protein: 15g

- Carbohydrates: 20g

- Fiber: 3g

- Potassium: 200mg

2. Apple Slices with Almond Butter

Ingredients:

- 1 apple, sliced
- Almond butter

Preparation:

1. Spread almond butter on apple slices.

Nutritional Information (per serving):

- Calories: 180
- Protein: 4g
- Carbohydrates: 25g
- Fiber: 6g
- Potassium: 180mg

3. Trail Mix

Ingredients:

- Almonds

- Walnuts

- Dried cranberries

- Dark chocolate chips

Preparation:

1. In a bowl, combine all the ingredients.

2. Portion into snack-sized bags.

Nutritional Information (per serving):

- Calories: 200

- Protein: 5g

- Carbohydrates: 15g

- Fiber: 4g

- Potassium: 150mg

4. Whole Grain Crackers with Cottage Cheese

Ingredients:

- Whole grain crackers
- Cottage cheese

Preparation:

1. Spread cottage cheese on whole grain crackers.

Nutritional Information (per serving):

- Calories: 120
- Protein: 8g
- Carbohydrates: 15g
- Fiber: 2g
- Potassium: 100mg

5. Cucumber and Tomato Salad

Ingredients:

- Cucumber, sliced

- Cherry tomatoes, halved

- Red onion, thinly sliced

- Olive oil

- Balsamic vinegar

- Fresh basil

- Salt and pepper to taste

Preparation:

1. Combine cucumber, tomatoes, and onion in a bowl.

2. Drizzle with balsamic vinegar and olive oil.

3. Sprinkle with fresh basil, salt, and pepper.

Nutritional Information (per serving):

- Calories: 80

- Protein: 2g

- Carbohydrates: 10g

- Fiber: 3g

- Potassium: 250mg

6. Roasted Chickpeas

Ingredients:

- Canned chickpeas, drained and rinsed

- Olive oil

- Smoked paprika

- Garlic powder

- Salt

Preparation:

1. Preheat oven to 400°F (200°C).

2. Toss chickpeas with olive oil, smoked paprika, garlic powder, and salt.

3. Roast in the oven until crispy, about 25-30 minutes.

Nutritional Information (per serving):

- Calories: 120

- Protein: 5g

- Carbohydrates: 15g

- Fiber: 5g

- Potassium: 180mg

7. Edamame

Ingredients:

- Edamame, steamed or boiled

- Sea salt

Preparation:

1. Sprinkle steamed or boiled edamame with sea salt.

Nutritional Information (per serving):

- Calories: 120

- Protein: 11g

- Carbohydrates: 8g

- Fiber: 4g

- Potassium: 370mg

8. Greek Salad Skewers

Ingredients:

- Cherry tomatoes

- Cucumber, cut into chunks

- Feta cheese, cubed

- Kalamata olives

- Olive oil

- Dried oregano

Preparation:

1. Skewer cherry tomatoes, cucumber, feta, and olives.

2. Drizzle with olive oil and sprinkle with dried oregano.

Nutritional Information (per serving):

- Calories: 100

- Protein: 3g

- Carbohydrates: 6g

- Fiber: 2g

- Potassium: 200mg

9. Avocado Toast

Ingredients:

- Whole grain bread

- Avocado, mashed

- Cherry tomatoes, sliced

- Salt and pepper to taste

Preparation:

1. Toast whole grain bread.

2. Spread mashed avocado on the toast.

3. Top with sliced cherry tomatoes.

4. Season with salt and pepper.

Nutritional Information (per serving):

- Calories: 180

- Protein: 5g

- Carbohydrates: 20g

- Fiber: 6g

- Potassium: 350mg

10. Quinoa Energy Balls

Ingredients:

- Cooked quinoa

- Almond butter

- Honey

- Chia seeds

- Dark chocolate chips

Preparation:

1. Mix quinoa, almond butter, honey, chia seeds, and chocolate chips in a bowl.

2. Form into small energy balls.

Nutritional Information (per serving):

- Calories: 150

- Protein: 4g

- Carbohydrates: 15g

- Fiber: 3g

- Potassium: 120mg

CHAPTER 9

Dessert Recipes

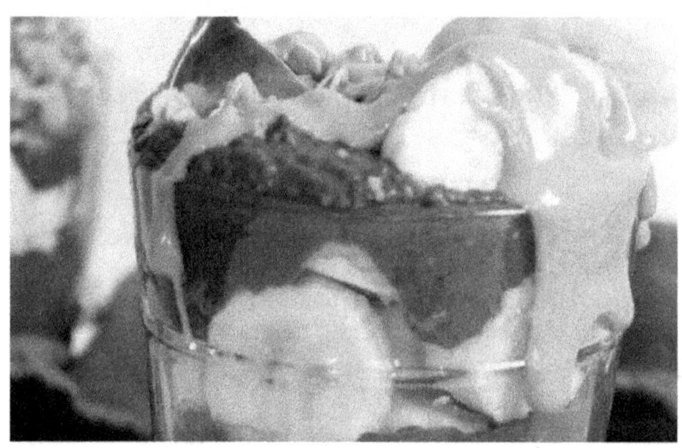

1. Chocolate Chia Pudding

Ingredients:

- Chia seeds

- Unsweetened cocoa powder

- Almond milk

- Maple syrup

- Vanilla extract

Preparation:

1. Mix chia seeds, cocoa powder, almond milk, maple syrup, and vanilla extract in a bowl.

2. Refrigerate overnight.

Nutritional Information (per serving):

- Calories: 120

- Protein: 4g

- Carbohydrates: 15g

- Fiber: 8g

- Potassium: 180mg

2. Sugar-Free Apple Tart

Ingredients:

- Whole wheat pie crust

- Apples, thinly sliced

- Cinnamon

- Stevia

Preparation:

1. Preheat oven to 375°F (190°C).

2. Arrange apple slices on the pie crust.

3. Sprinkle with cinnamon and stevia.

4. Bake until apples are tender, about 25 minutes.

Nutritional Information (per serving):

- Calories: 140

- Protein: 2g

- Carbohydrates: 30g

- Fiber: 5g

- Potassium: 150mg

3. Strawberry Panna Cotta

Ingredients:

- Greek yogurt

- Strawberries, pureed

- Gelatin

- Honey

- Vanilla extract

Preparation:

1. Bloom gelatin in cold water, then dissolve in warm water.

2. Mix yogurt, strawberry puree, honey, and vanilla.

3. Add dissolved gelatin and pour into molds.

4. Refrigerate until set.

Nutritional Information (per serving):

- Calories: 110

- Protein: 8g

- Carbohydrates: 15g

- Fiber: 2g

- Potassium: 200mg

4. Banana Ice Cream

Ingredients:

- Bananas, sliced and frozen

- Almond milk

- Vanilla extract

Preparation:

1. Blend frozen bananas, almond milk, and vanilla extract until creamy.

2. Freeze for a firmer texture.

Nutritional Information (per serving):

- Calories: 100

- Protein: 1g

- Carbohydrates: 25g

- Fiber: 3g

- Potassium: 400mg

5. Oatmeal Raisin Cookies

Ingredients:

- Rolled oats

- Whole wheat flour

- Raisins

- Coconut oil

- Maple syrup

Preparation:

1. Mix oats, flour, raisins, coconut oil, and maple syrup.

2. Form into cookies and bake at 350°F (180°C) for 12-15 minutes.

Nutritional Information (per serving):

- Calories: 90

- Protein: 2g

- Carbohydrates: 15g

- Fiber: 2g

- Potassium: 110mg

6. Coconut Tapioca Pudding

Ingredients:

- Tapioca pearls

- Coconut milk

- Stevia

- Coconut flakes

Preparation:

1. Cook tapioca pearls in coconut milk until translucent.

2. Sweeten with stevia, chill, and top with coconut flakes.

Nutritional Information (per serving):

- Calories: 130

- Protein: 1g

- Carbohydrates: 25g

- Fiber: 1g

- Potassium: 90mg

7. Almond Butter Cookies

- Almond butter

- Oat flour

- Almond flour

- Maple syrup

- Vanilla extract

1. Mix almond butter, oat flour, almond flour, maple syrup, and vanilla.

2. Form into cookies and bake at 350°F (180°C) for 10-12 minutes.

Nutritional Information (per serving):

- Calories: 110

- Protein: 3g

- Carbohydrates: 10g

- Fiber: 2g

- Potassium: 70mg

8. Berry Parfait

Ingredients:

- Mixed berries

- Greek yogurt

- Granola

- Honey

Preparation:

1. Layer berries, yogurt, granola, and drizzle with honey.

Nutritional Information (per serving):

- Calories: 150

- Protein: 6g

- Carbohydrates: 25g

- Fiber: 5g

- Potassium: 220mg

9. Chocolate Avocado Mousse

Ingredients:

- Avocado

- Unsweetened cocoa powder

- Maple syrup

- Vanilla extract

Preparation:

1. Blend avocado, cocoa powder, maple syrup, and vanilla until smooth.

2. Chill before serving.

Nutritional Information (per serving):

- Calories: 130

- Protein: 2g

- Carbohydrates: 15g

- Fiber: 5g

- Potassium: 290mg

10. Vanilla Chia Pudding

- Chia seeds

- Almond milk

- Vanilla extract

- Honey

Preparation:

1. Mix chia seeds, almond milk, vanilla extract, and honey.

2. Refrigerate until pudding-like consistency.

Nutritional Information (per serving):

- Calories: 120

- Protein: 4g

- Carbohydrates: 15g

- Fiber: 8g

- Potassium: 180mg

30 Day Meal Plan

Week 1

Day 1:

Breakfast: Blueberry Oatmeal

Lunch: Chicken and Vegetable Stir Fry

Dinner: Quinoa Stuffed Bell Pepper

Snack: Greek Yogurt with Berries

Dessert: Chocolate Chia Pudding

Day 2:

Breakfast: Scrambled Egg and Vegetables

Lunch: Turkey and Vegetable Chili

Dinner: Lemon Herb Grilled Chicken Breast

Snack: Apple Slices with Almond Butter

Dessert: Sugar-Free Apple Tart

Day 3:

Breakfast: Avocado and Egg Toast

Lunch: Grilled Lemon Herb Chicken

Dinner: Baked Cod with Roasted Vegetables

Snack: Trail Mix

Dessert: Strawberry Panna Cotta

Day 4:

Breakfast: Veggie Omelet

Lunch: Greek-Style Quinoa Salad

Dinner: Chickpea and Vegetable Curry

Snack: Whole Grain Crackers with Cottage Cheese

Dessert: Banana Ice Cream

Day 5:

Breakfast: Pineapple Coconut Smoothie

Lunch: Grilled Chicken Quinoa Salad

Dinner: Caprese Stuffed Chicken Breast

Snack: Cucumber and Tomato Salad

Dessert: Oatmeal Raisin Cookies

Day 6:

Breakfast: Chia Seed Pudding

Lunch: Baked Salmon with Lemon and Dill

Dinner: Baked Zucchini Boats with Ground Turkey

Snack: Roasted Chickpeas

Dessert: Coconut Tapioca Pudding

Day 7:

Breakfast: Quinoa Breakfast Porridge

Lunch: Chicken Curry with Vegetables

Dinner: Spicy Shrimp Stir Fry with Brown Rice

Snack: Edamame

Dessert: Almond Butter Cookies

Week 2

Day 8:

Breakfast: Avocado and Egg Toast

Lunch: Grilled Lemon Herb Chicken

Dinner: Baked Cod with Roasted Vegetables

Snack: Trail Mix

Dessert: Strawberry Panna Cotta

Day 9:

Breakfast: Veggie Omelet

Lunch: Greek-Style Quinoa Salad

Dinner: Chickpea and Vegetable Curry

Snack: Whole Grain Crackers with Cottage Cheese

Dessert: Banana Ice Cream

Day 10:

Breakfast: Pineapple Coconut Smoothie

Lunch: Grilled Chicken Quinoa Salad

Dinner: Caprese Stuffed Chicken Breast

Snack: Cucumber and Tomato Salad

Dessert: Oatmeal Raisin Cookies

Day 11:

Breakfast: Blueberry Oatmeal

Lunch: Chicken and Vegetable Stir Fry

Dinner: Quinoa Stuffed Bell Pepper

Snack: Greek Yogurt with Berries

Dessert: Chocolate Chia Pudding

Day 12:

Breakfast: Scrambled Egg and Vegetables

Lunch: Turkey and Vegetable Chili

Dinner: Lemon Herb Grilled Chicken Breast

Snack: Apple Slices with Almond Butter

Dessert: Sugar-Free Apple Tart

Day 13:

Breakfast: Quinoa Breakfast Porridge

Lunch: Chicken Curry with Vegetables

Dinner: Spicy Shrimp Stir Fry with Brown Rice

Snack: Edamame

Dessert: Almond Butter Cookies

Day 14:

Breakfast: Chia Seed Pudding

Lunch: Baked Salmon with Lemon and Dill

Dinner: Baked Zucchini Boats with Ground Turkey

Snack: Roasted Chickpeas

Dessert: Coconut Tapioca Pudding

Week 3

Day 15:

Breakfast: Avocado and Egg Toast

Lunch: Grilled Lemon Herb Chicken

Dinner: Baked Cod with Roasted Vegetables

Snack: Trail Mix

Dessert: Strawberry Panna Cotta

Day 16:

Breakfast: Blueberry Oatmeal

Lunch: Chicken and Vegetable Stir Fry

Dinner: Quinoa Stuffed Bell Pepper

Snack: Greek Yogurt with Berries

Dessert: Chocolate Chia Pudding

Day 17:

Breakfast: Scrambled Egg and Vegetables

Lunch: Turkey and Vegetable Chili

Dinner: Lemon Herb Grilled Chicken Breast

Snack: Apple Slices with Almond Butter

Dessert: Sugar-Free Apple Tart

Day 18:

Breakfast: Quinoa Breakfast Porridge

Lunch: Chicken Curry with Vegetables

Dinner: Spicy Shrimp Stir Fry with Brown Rice

Snack: Edamame

Dessert: Almond Butter Cookies

Day 19:

Breakfast: Blueberry Oatmeal

Lunch: Chicken and Vegetable Stir Fry

Dinner: Quinoa Stuffed Bell Pepper

Snack: Greek Yogurt with Berries

Dessert: Chocolate Chia Pudding

Day 20:

Breakfast: Scrambled Egg and Vegetables

Lunch: Turkey and Vegetable Chili

Dinner: Lemon Herb Grilled Chicken Breast

Snack: Apple Slices with Almond Butter

Dessert: Sugar-Free Apple Tart

Day 21:

Breakfast: Avocado and Egg Toast

Lunch: Grilled Lemon Herb Chicken

Dinner: Baked Cod with Roasted Vegetables

Snack: Trail Mix

Dessert: Strawberry Panna Cotta

Week 4

Breakfast: Veggie Omelet

Lunch: Greek-Style Quinoa Salad

Dinner: Chickpea and Vegetable Curry

Snack: Whole Grain Crackers with Cottage Cheese

Dessert: Banana Ice Cream

Breakfast: Pineapple Coconut Smoothie

Lunch: Grilled Chicken Quinoa Salad

Dinner: Caprese Stuffed Chicken Breast

Snack: Cucumber and Tomato Salad

Dessert: Oatmeal Raisin Cookies

Day 24:

Breakfast: Chia Seed Pudding

Lunch: Baked Salmon with Lemon and Dill

Dinner: Baked Zucchini Boats with Ground Turkey

Snack: Roasted Chickpeas

Dessert: Coconut Tapioca Pudding

Day 25:

Breakfast: Quinoa Breakfast Porridge

Lunch: Chicken Curry with Vegetables

Dinner: Spicy Shrimp Stir Fry with Brown Rice

Snack: Edamame

Dessert: Almond Butter Cookies

Day 26:

Breakfast: Scrambled Egg and Vegetables

Lunch: Turkey and Vegetable Chili

Dinner: Lemon Herb Grilled Chicken Breast

Snack: Apple Slices with Almond Butter

Dessert: Sugar-Free Apple Tart

Day 27:

Breakfast: Avocado and Egg Toast

Lunch: Grilled Lemon Herb Chicken

Dinner: Baked Cod with Roasted Vegetables

Snack: Trail Mix

Dessert: Strawberry Panna Cotta

Day 28:

Breakfast: Pineapple Coconut Smoothie

Lunch: Grilled Chicken Quinoa Salad

Dinner: Caprese Stuffed Chicken Breast

Snack: Cucumber and Tomato Salad

Dessert: Oatmeal Raisin Cookies

Day 29:

Breakfast: Chia Seed Pudding

Lunch: Baked Salmon with Lemon and Dill

Dinner: Baked Zucchini Boats with Ground Turkey

Snack: Roasted Chickpeas

Dessert: Coconut Tapioca Pudding

Day 30:

Breakfast: Quinoa Breakfast Porridge

Lunch: Chicken Curry with Vegetables

Dinner: Spicy Shrimp Stir Fry with Brown Rice

Snack: Edamame

Dessert: Almond Butter Cookies

CONCLUSION

Finally, I would like to express my sincere gratitude for starting this journey toward a healthier lifestyle with the Dash Diet Cookbook for Beginners 2024. This dietary approach has endless benefits, and you deserve praise for your dedication to putting your health first.

You have not only fed your body with the variety and delicious recipes in this cookbook, but you have also developed a new relationship with food that supports heart health, improves general wellbeing, and gives life more energy.

Recall that following the Dash Diet is a commitment to your own well-being, a path to a vibrant future, and more than just a food decision. You have the ability to change your life, and every nutritious meal you eat is an investment in a happier, healthier you.

This is your unique motivation, so enjoy every wholesome bite, welcome this journey with joy, and bask in the positive changes that will undoubtedly occur. You will receive gratitude from your heart, your body, and your future self.

As you continue down this path toward wellness, may the flavors of these Dash Diet recipes uplift and delight you, and may your dedication to well-being be the driving force behind each and every culinary decision. You've made a big step in the right direction.

Here's to you, your health, and the vibrant future that lies ahead. Stay inspired, stay committed, and savor the journey to a heart-healthy and fulfilling life!

My Little Request

Dear Reader,

Thanks for your purchase, hope you enjoyed reading.

Could you please take a few seconds to leave a positive feedback on this book?

It'll help reach more people and we can collectively help reverse this deadly disease.

Thank you.

BONUS: WEEKLY MEAL PLANNER JOURNAL

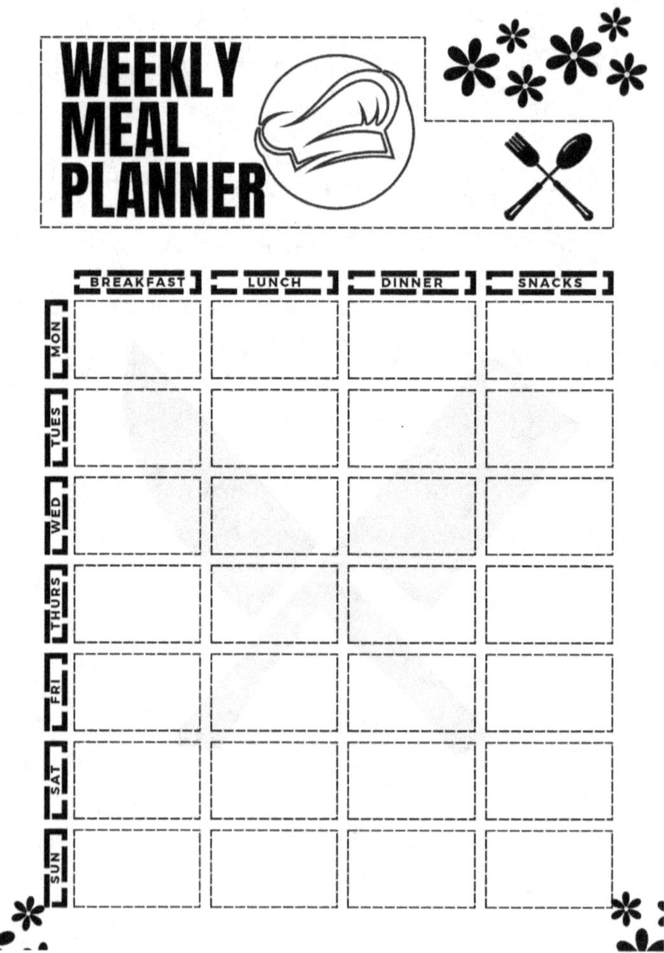

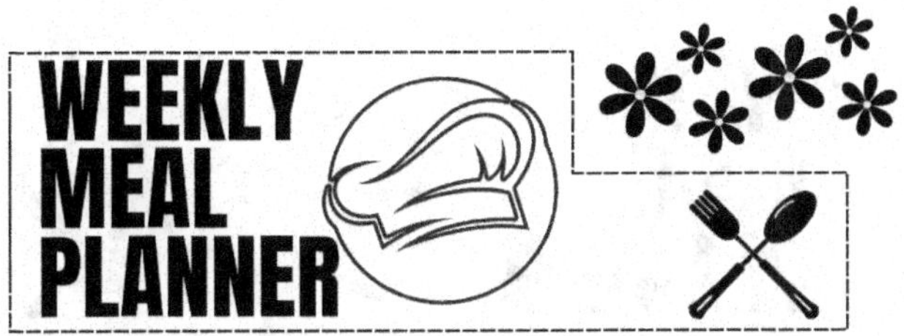

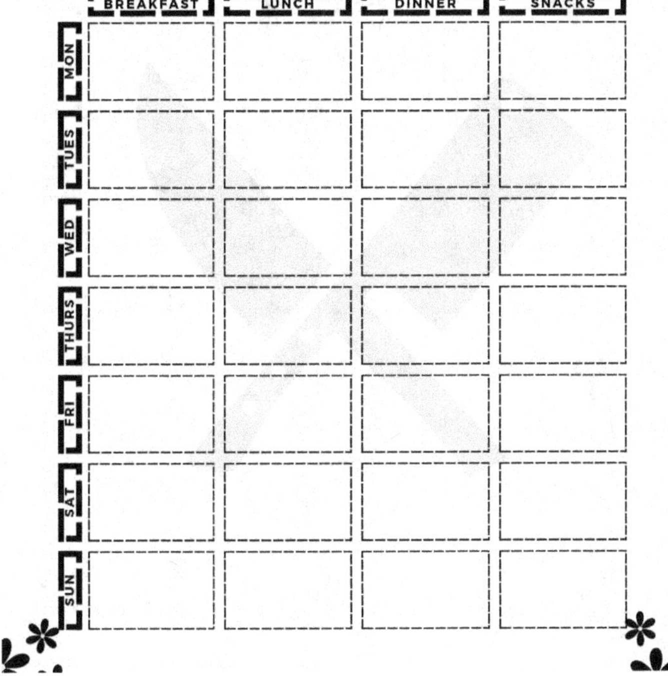

BREAKFAST
LUNCH
DINNER
SNACKS
MON
TUES
WED
THURS
FRI
SAT
SUN

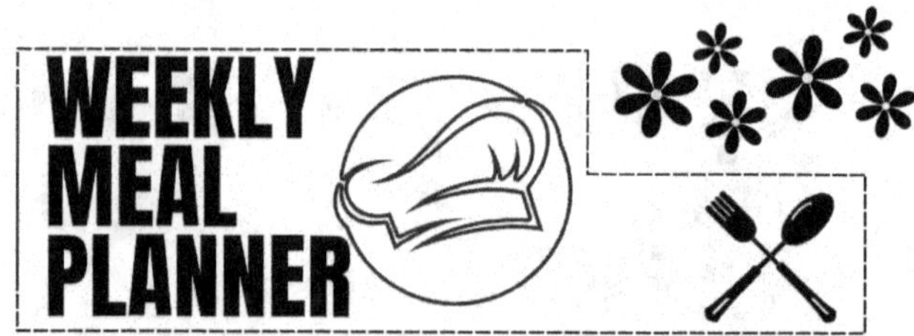

WEEKLY
MEAL
PLANNER

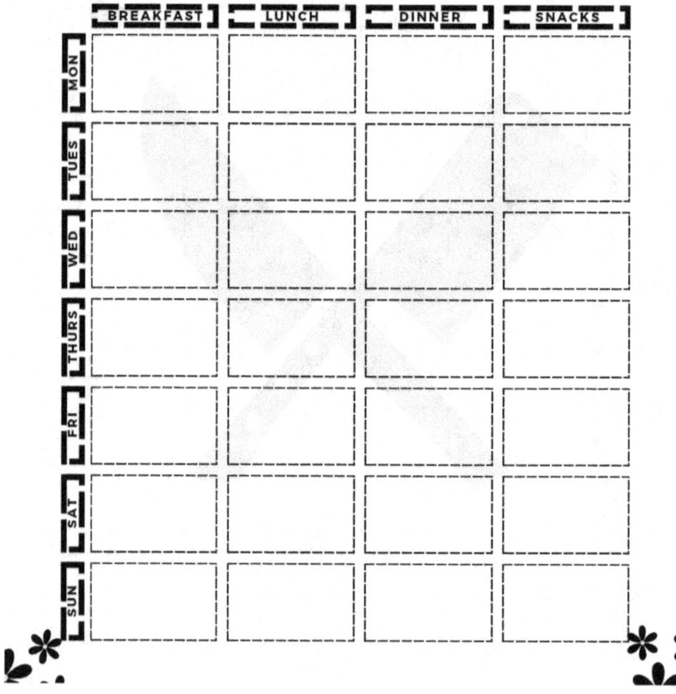

BREAKFAST
LUNCH
DINNER
SNACKS
MON
TUES
WED
THURS
FRI
SAT
SUN

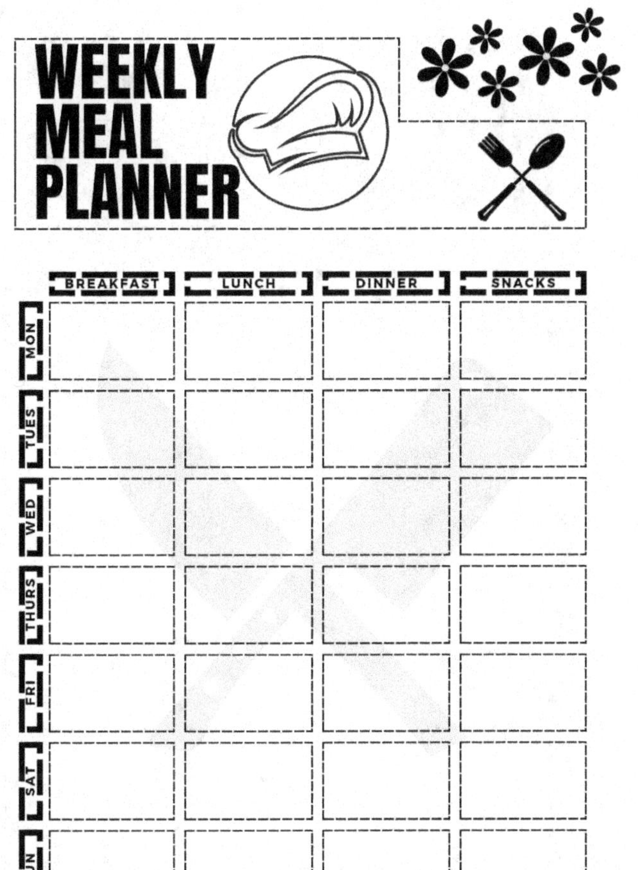

WEEKLY
MEAL
PLANNER
BREAKFAST
LUNCH
DINNER
SNACKS
MON
TUES
WED
THURS
FRI
SAT
SUN

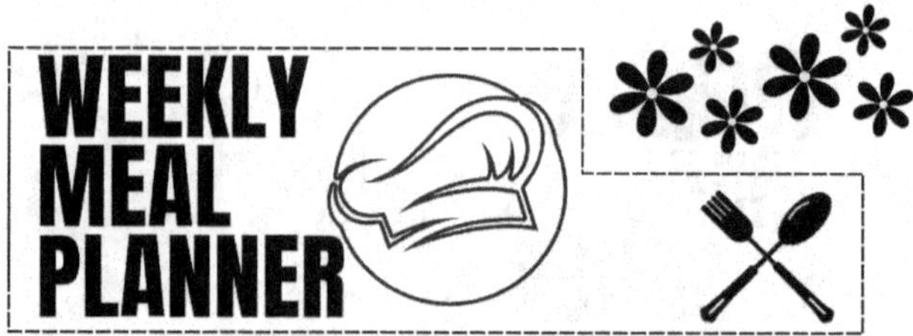

WEEKLY
MEAL
PLANNER

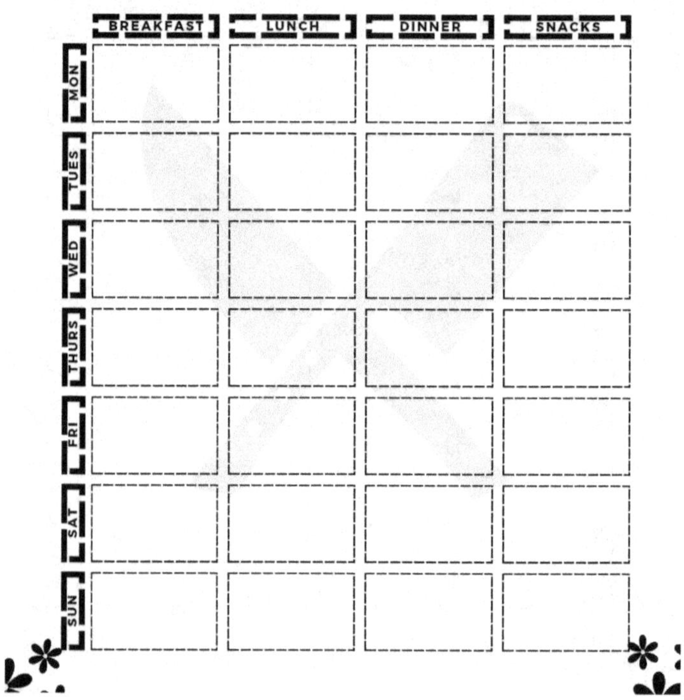

BREAKFAST
LUNCH
DINNER
SNACKS
MON
TUES
WED
THURS
FRI
SAT
SUN

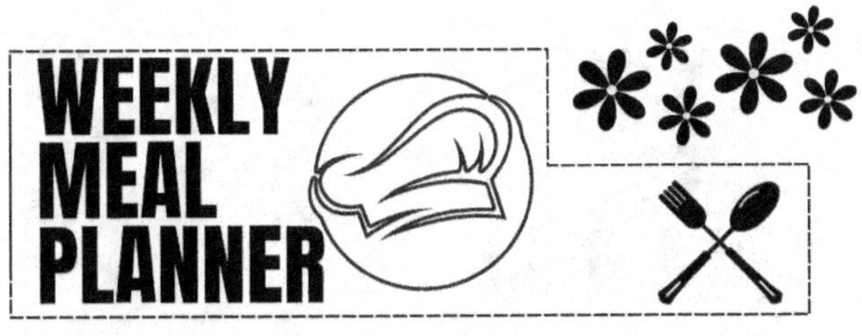

	BREAKFAST	LUNCH	DINNER	SNACKS
MON				
TUES				
WED				
THURS				
FRI				
SAT				
SUN				

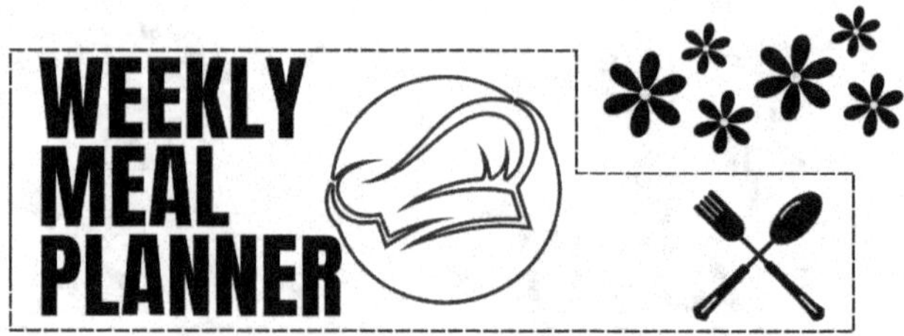

WEEKLY
MEAL
PLANNER

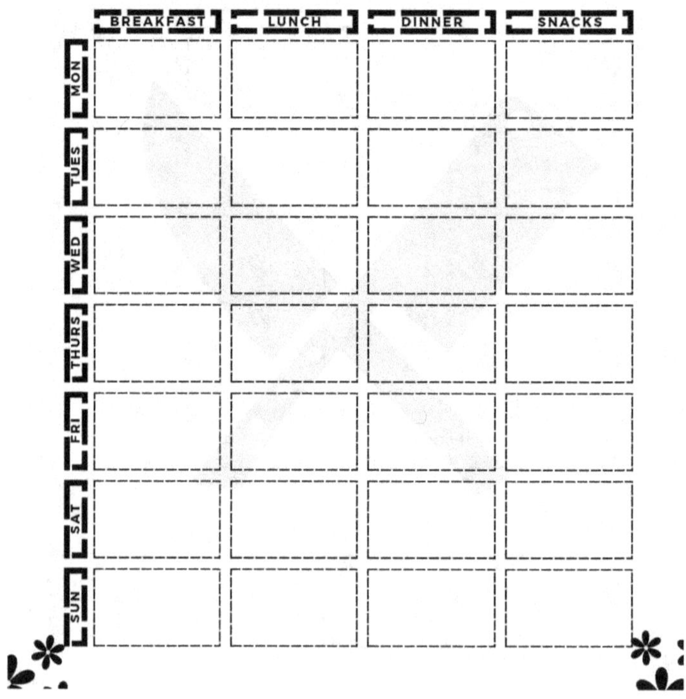

BREAKFAST
LUNCH
DINNER
SNACKS
MON
TUES
WED
THURS
FRI
SAT
SUN

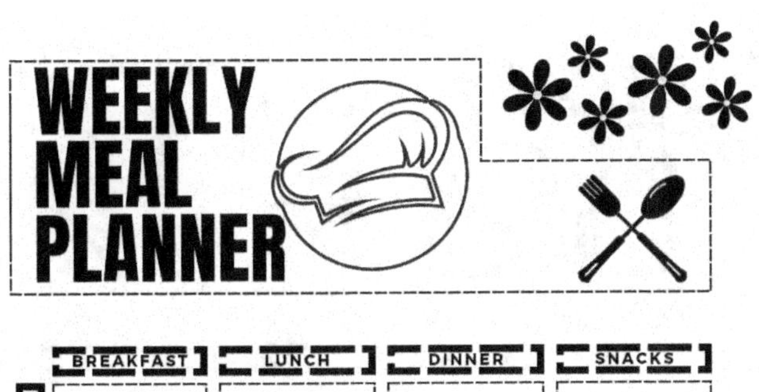

WEEKLY
MEAL
PLANNER

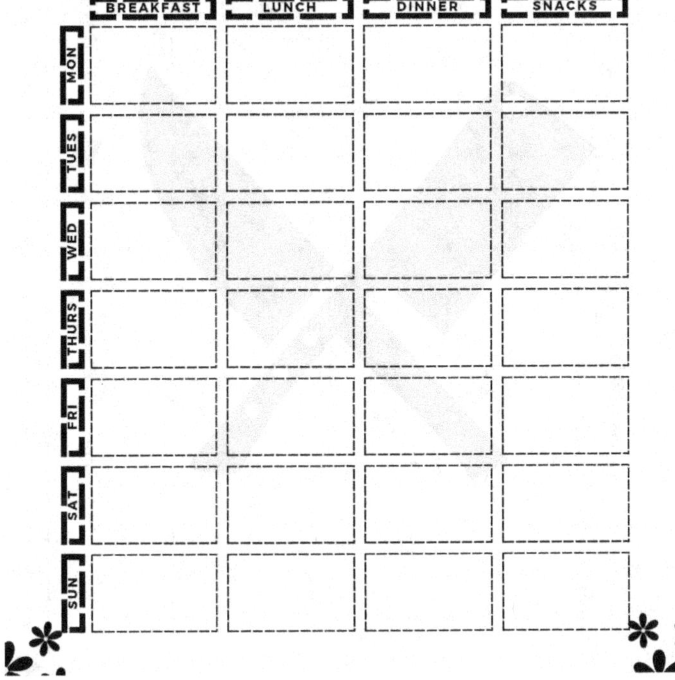

BREAKFAST
LUNCH
DINNER
SNACKS
MON
TUES
WED
THURS
FRI
SAT
SUN

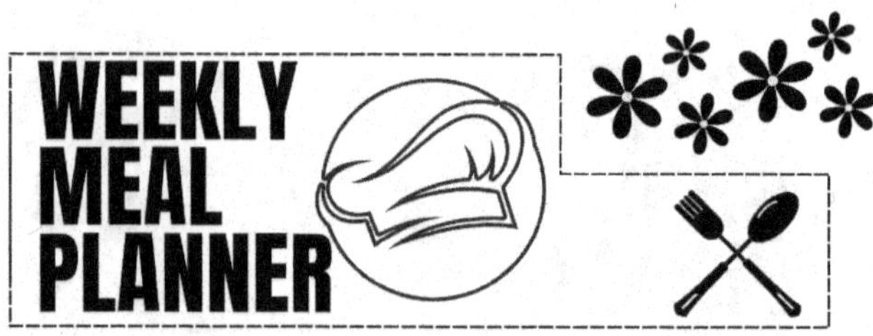

WEEKLY
MEAL
PLANNER

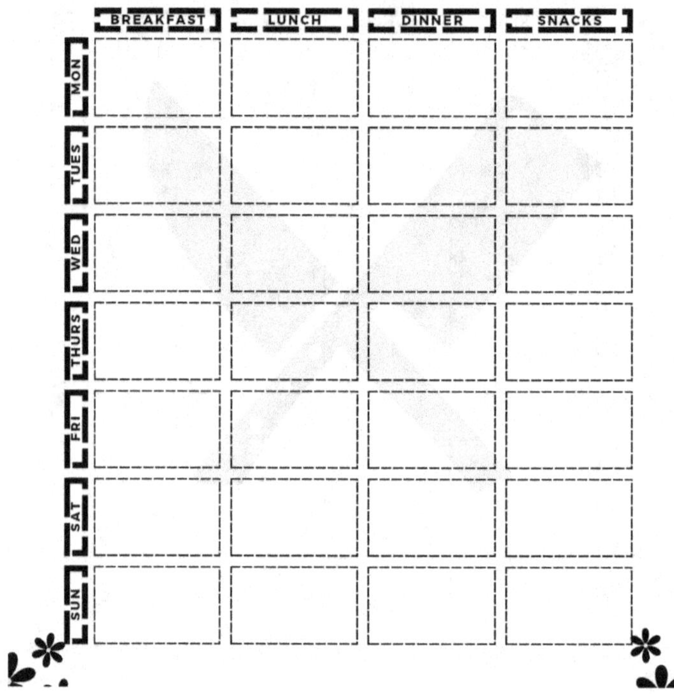

BREAKFAST
LUNCH
DINNER
SNACKS
MON
TUES
WED
THURS
FRI
SAT
SUN

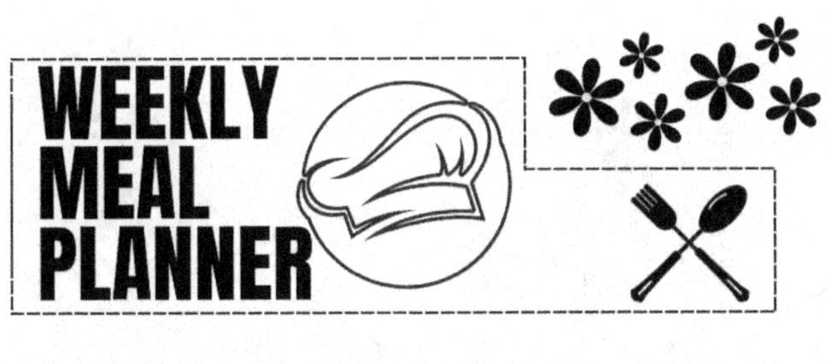

WEEKLY
MEAL
PLANNER

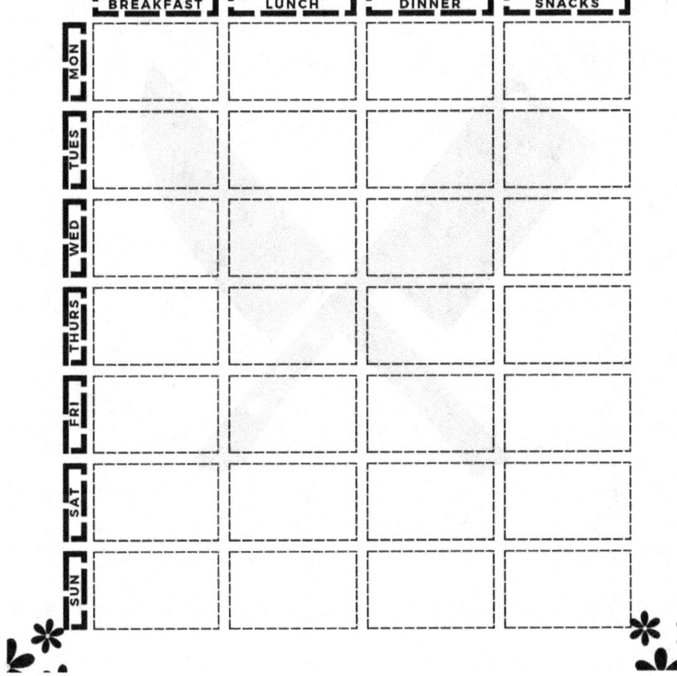

BREAKFAST
LUNCH
DINNER
SNACKS
MON
TUES
WED
THURS
FRI
SAT
SUN

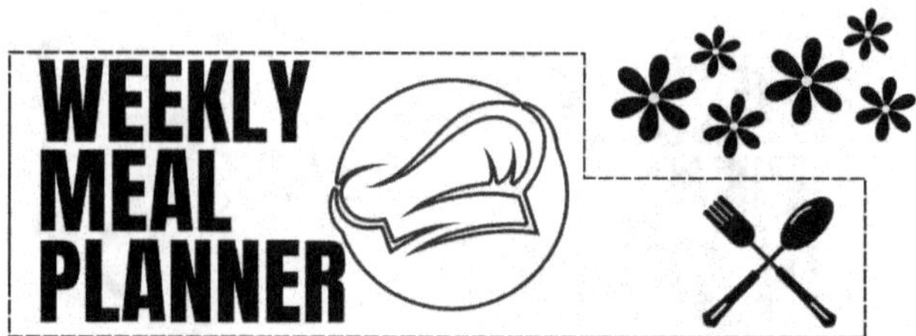

WEEKLY
MEAL
PLANNER

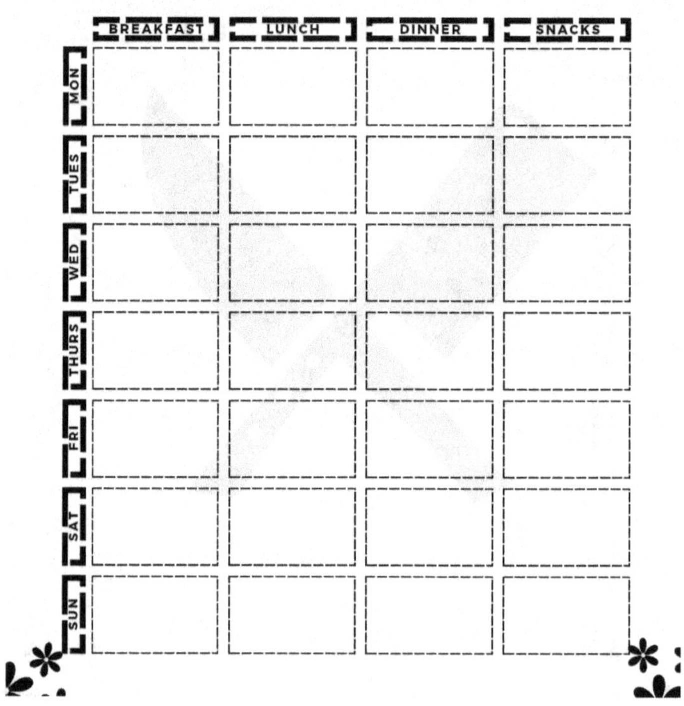

BREAKFAST
LUNCH
DINNER
SNACKS
MON
TUES
WED
THURS
FRI
SAT
SUN

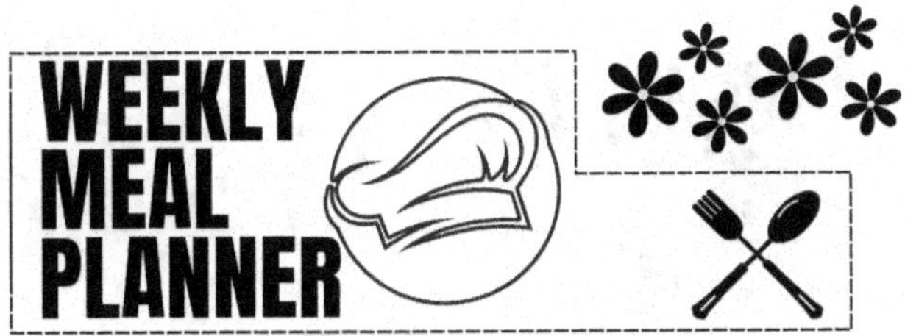

	BREAKFAST	LUNCH	DINNER	SNACKS
MON				
TUES				
WED				
THURS				
FRI				
SAT				
SUN				

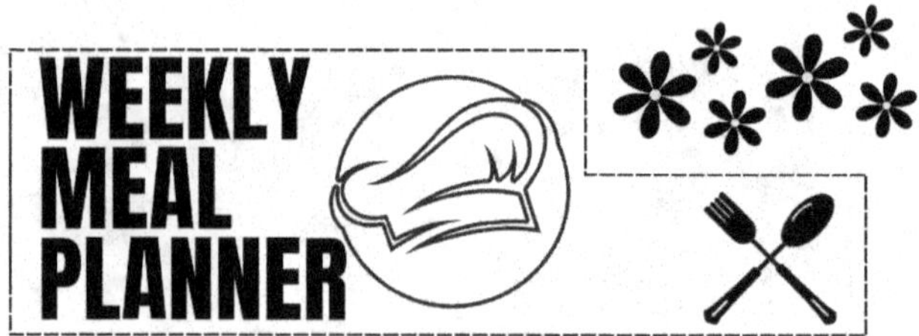

WEEKLY
MEAL
PLANNER

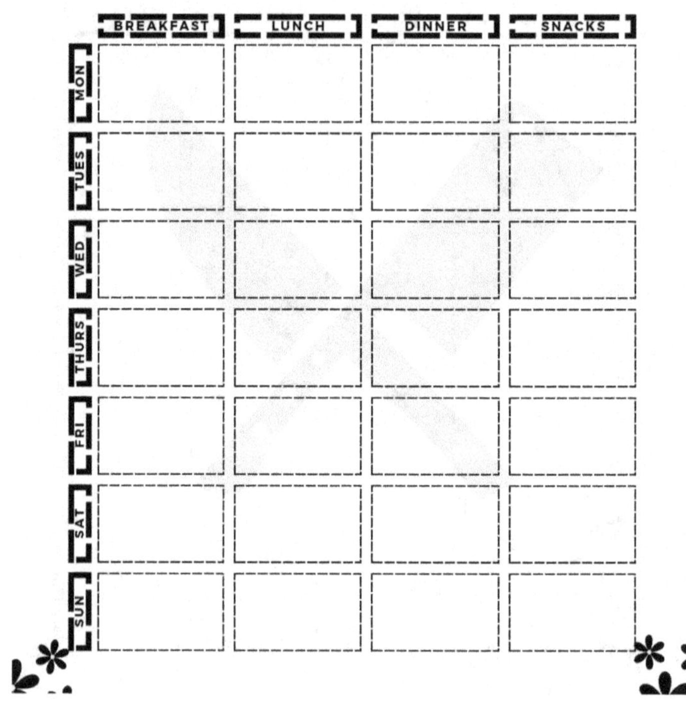

BREAKFAST
LUNCH
DINNER
SNACKS
MON
TUES
WED
THURS
FRI
SAT
SUN

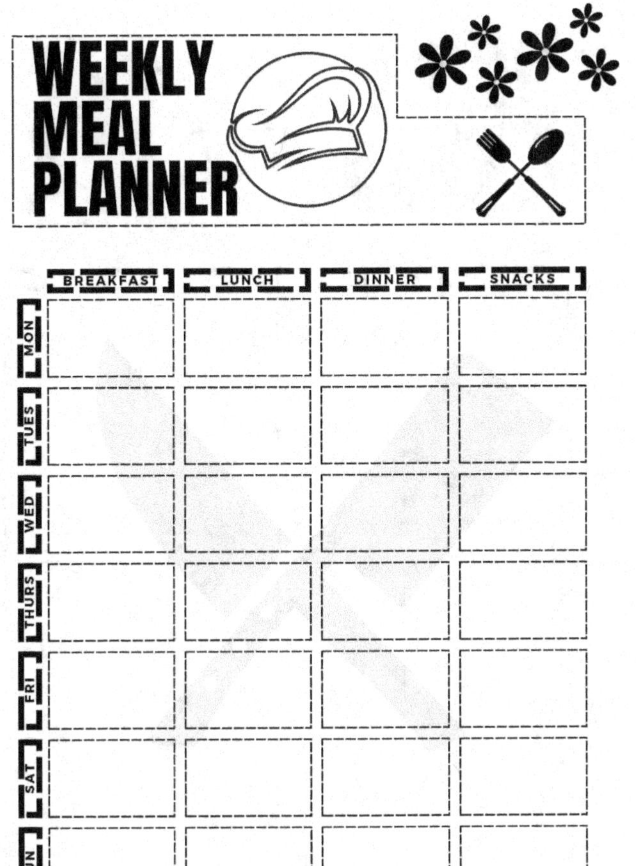

WEEKLY MEAL PLANNER
BREAKFAST
LUNCH
DINNER
SNACKS
MON
TUES
WED
THURS
FRI
SAT
SUN

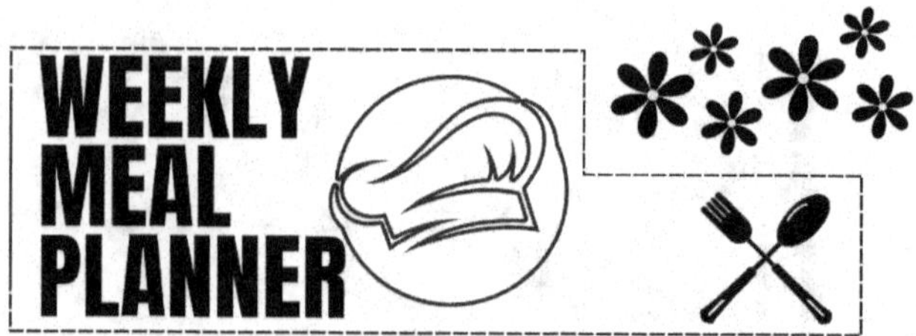

WEEKLY
MEAL
PLANNER

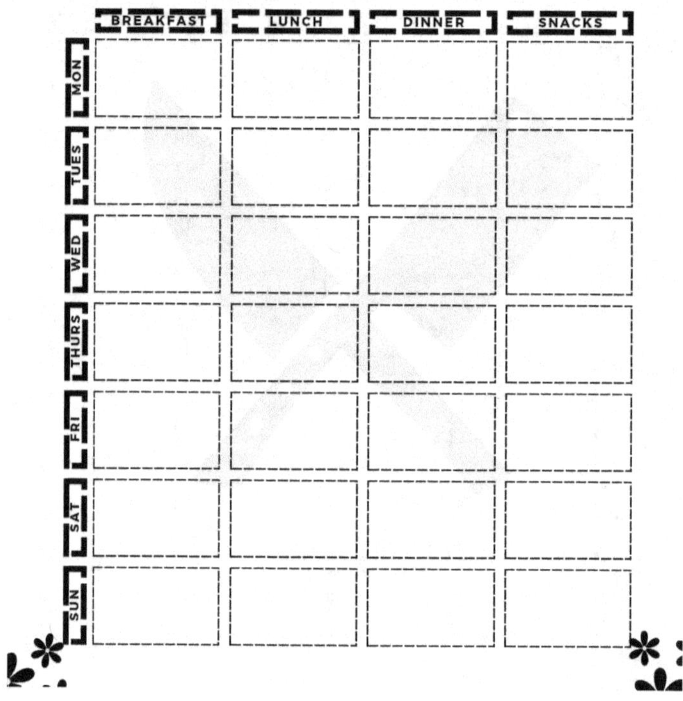

BREAKFAST
LUNCH
DINNER
SNACKS
MON
TUES
WED
THURS
FRI
SAT
SUN

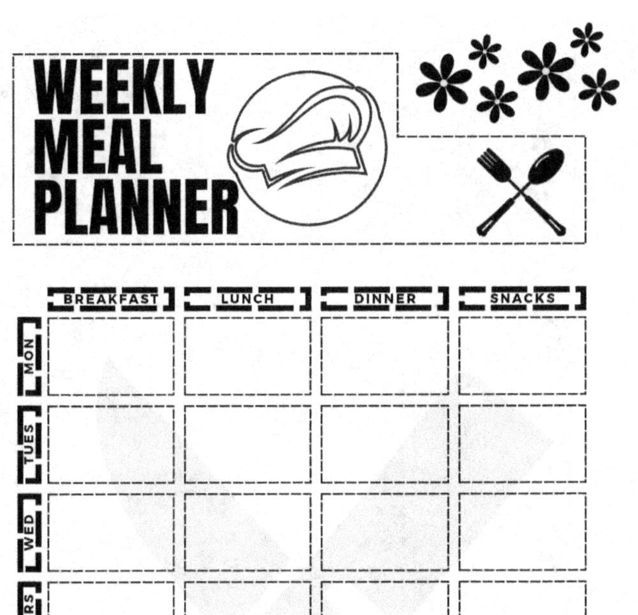

WEEKLY MEAL PLANNER
BREAKFAST
LUNCH
DINNER
SNACKS
MON
TUES
WED
THURS
FRI
SAT
SUN

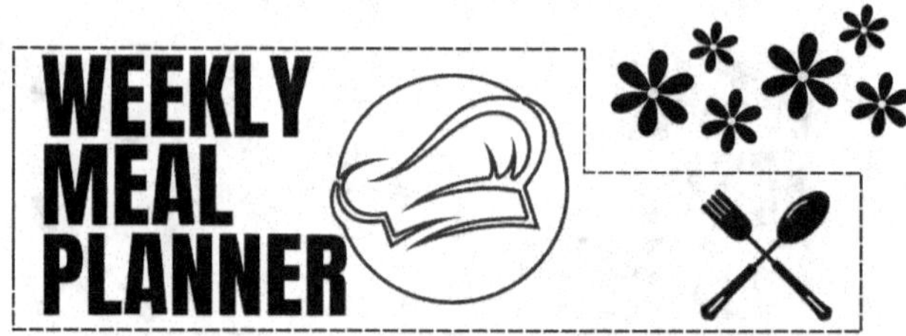

WEEKLY
MEAL
PLANNER

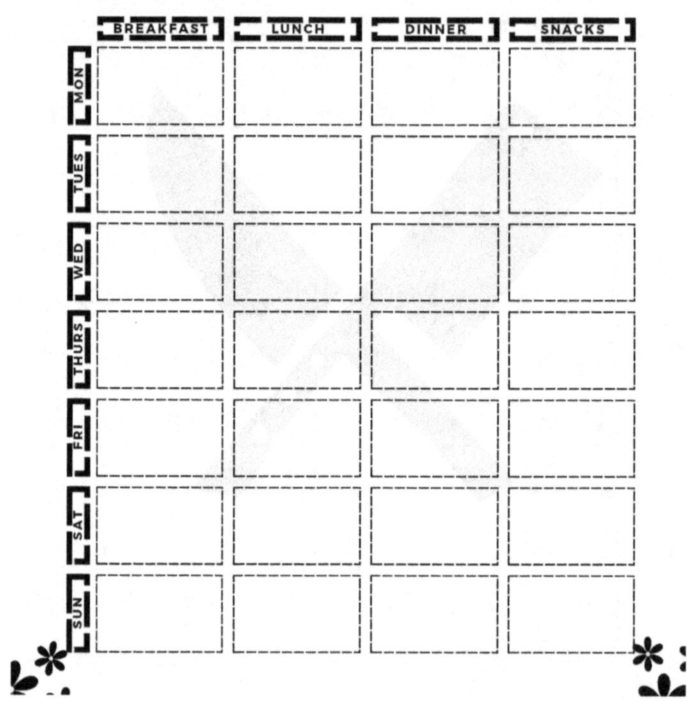

BREAKFAST
LUNCH
DINNER
SNACKS
MON
TUES
WED
THURS
FRI
SAT
SUN

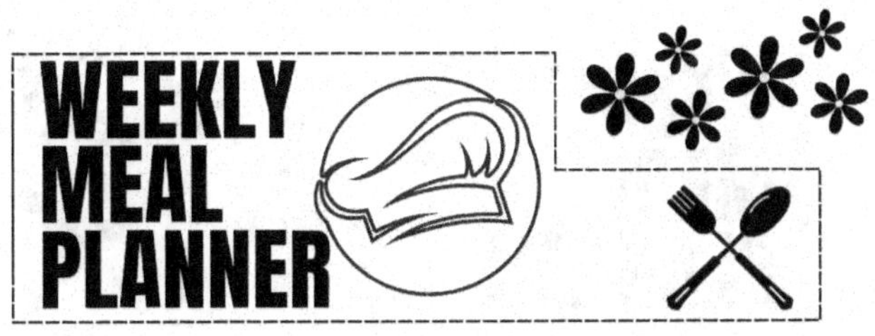

WEEKLY
MEAL
PLANNER

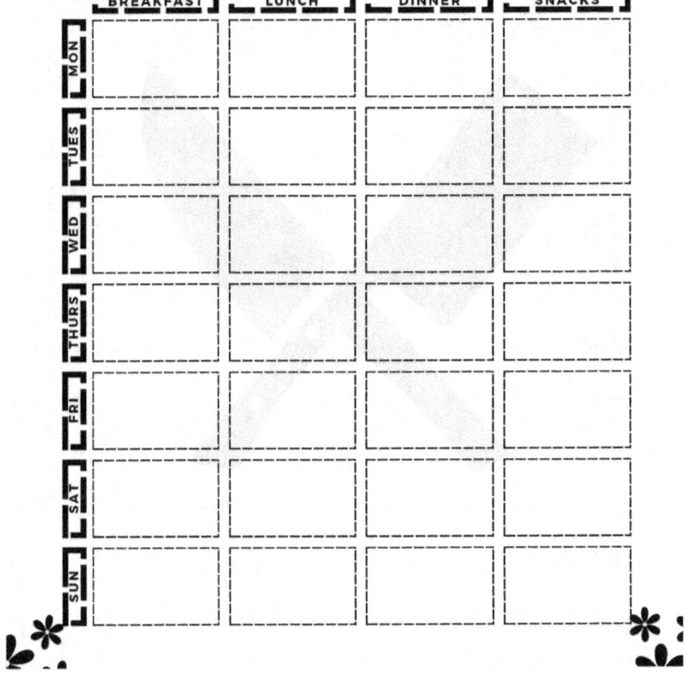

BREAKFAST
LUNCH
DINNER
SNACKS
MON
TUES
WED
THURS
FRI
SAT
SUN

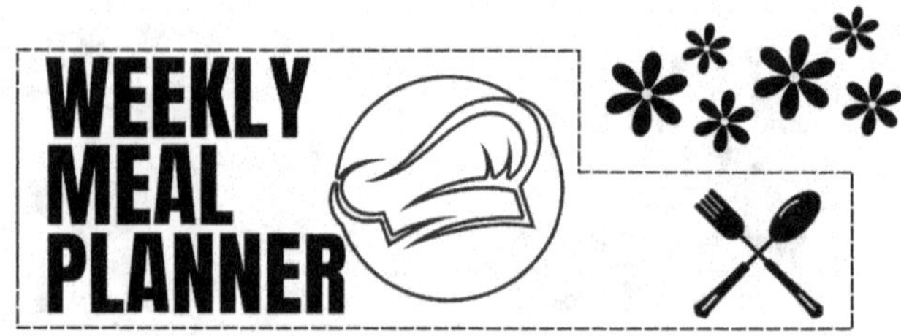

WEEKLY
MEAL
PLANNER

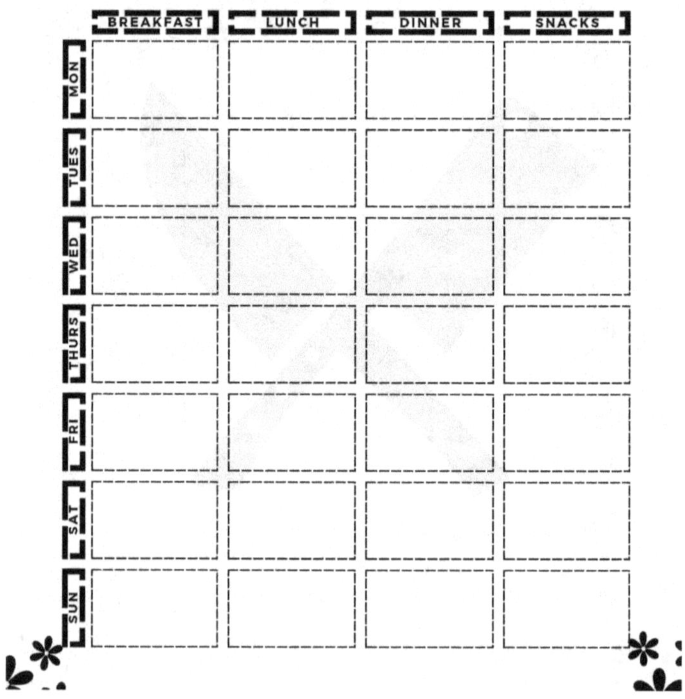

BREAKFAST
LUNCH
DINNER
SNACKS
MON
TUES
WED
THURS
FRI
SAT
SUN

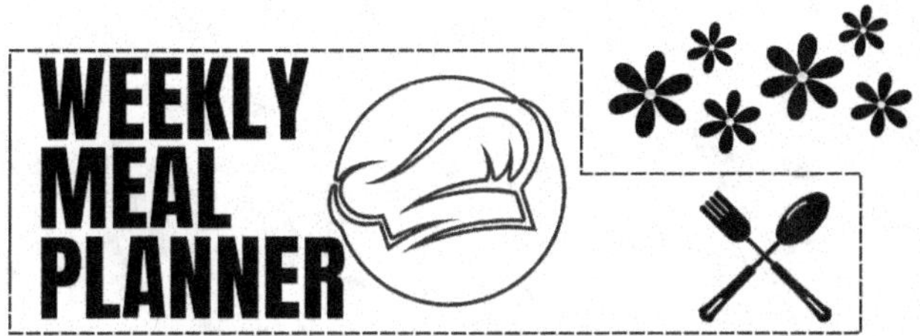

WEEKLY
MEAL
PLANNER

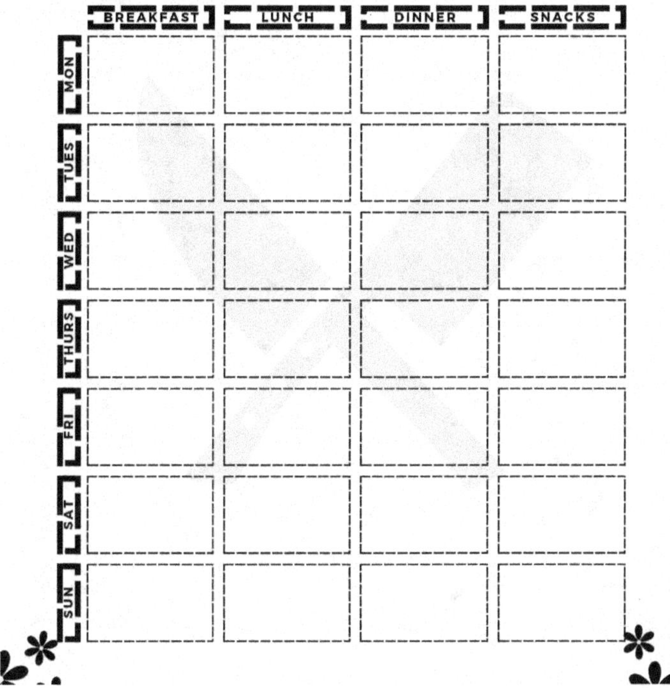

BREAKFAST
LUNCH
DINNER
SNACKS
MON
TUES
WED
THURS
FRI
SAT
SUN

www.ingramcontent.com/pod-product-compliance
Lightning Source LLC
Chambersburg PA
CBHW070930260726
48661CB00003B/915